Health Care Fraud: A Prescription for Disaster

William E. Ackerman MD

Health Care Fraud: A Prescription for Disaster

Copyright © 2017 by William E. Ackerman MD

All rights reserved. No part of this book may be reproduced or transmitted in any form or by any means without written permission of the author.

I dedicate this book to my children and grandchildren that they may have adequate health care in the future.

Acknowledgments

I acknowledge my patients who were kind enough to share some of their health care fraud stories with me.

Foreword

No doctor wants to be identified as being out of step with medical practice norms. Furthermore, most health care providers do not want a decrease in profit margins as well. This book is about the millions of Americans who have access to what some would call the best medical care in the world but are being defrauded. Of course, there are millions of uninsured Americans whose access to care is heartlessly limited. The problems of fraudulent health care described in this book are less likely to transpire to the latter group, simply because they receive less medical care.

This book is about the relentless expansion of medicine and our health providers increasing tendency to only make a diagnosis so that further treatments can be done to increase their revenues. Americans have been taught to be concerned about their health. We are all aware that types of hidden jeopardies prowl inside of us. The conventional wisdom is that it's always better to know about these dangers so that something can be done. That's why we are so enthusiastic about amazing medical technologies that can detect abnormalities even when we reason we are well. That's also why we welcome the identification of risk factors, disease awareness campaigns, cancer screening, genetic testing etc. Americans love a diagnosis so that they can receive attention and health care whether or not it helps them. But it's also true that we do receive too much of it in some circumstances. Some people are diagnosed and treated needlessly by swindlers who do unnecessary or dangerous treatments to increase their profit which is one reason why this book was written. Another reason for this book is to inform individuals that rewards can be made by reporting health care fraud by becoming a whistle blower. Health care consumers need to identify these health care fraudsters and report them to ultimately attempt to salvage what remains of our health care structure. Health deception costs Americans billions of dollars. We all must do our parts to reverse this trend including health care professionals. Voltaire once stated: "Doctors are men who prescribe medicines of which they know little, to cure diseases of which they know less, in human beings of whom they know nothing."

Table of Contents

1. Health Care Fraud 1
2. Health Care Fraud is a Crime 7
3. Whistleblowers 15
4. Health Provider Fraud 25
5. Hospital Fraud 31
6. Medical Necessity Fraud 39
7. Pharmaceutical Company Fraud 43
8. Medical Transport Fraud 51
9. Workman's Compensation Fraud 57
10. Pill Mill Fraud 65
11. Addiction Medicine Fraud 73
12. Medical Laboratory Fraud 81
13. Pharmacy Fraud 89
14. Compound Drug Fraud 95
15. Alternative Medicine Fraud 103
16. Drug Cost Fraud 111
17. Optometry Fraud 117
18. Chiropractic Fraud 123
19. Medical Research Fraud 131
20. Dentistry Fraud 135
21. Podiatry Fraud 139
22. Nurse Fraud 143
23. Physical Therapy Fraud 149
24. Occupational Therapy Fraud 155

25. Allergist Fraud 163

26. Anesthesia Fraud 169

27. Cosmetic Surgery Fraud 175

28. Cardiology Fraud 181

29. Dermatology Fraud 187

30. Emergency Medicine Fraud 195

31. Endocrinology Fraud 203

32. Family Practice Fraud 205

33. Gastroenterology Fraud 211

34. Geriatrics Fraud 217

35. Infectious Disease Fraud 225

36. Internal Medicine Fraud 231

37. Kidney Disease Fraud 235

38. Neurology Fraud 241

39. Neurosurgery Fraud 249

40. Obstetrics Gynecology Fraud 255

41. Oncology Fraud 261

42. Ophthalmology Fraud 267

43. Orthopedic Surgery Fraud 273

44. Otolaryngology Fraud 279

45. Pain Management Fraud 283

46. Palliative Care Fraud 289

47. Pathology Fraud 295

48. Pediatric Fraud 299

49. Physical Medicine Fraud 305

50. Psychiatry Fraud 309

51. Pulmonology Fraud 315
52. Radiology Fraud 323
53. Urology Fraud 329
54. Virology Fraud 333

1. Health Care Fraud

The medical profession and health care in general has deteriorated over the past twenty years. It has become plagued with fraudulent behaviors. It is difficult for individuals to know if they are being scammed. Fraud unfortunately exists in all aspects of health care today.

Fraud means an intentional deception or misrepresentation made by a person with the knowledge that the deception could result in some unauthorized benefit to himself or some other person." "Abuse means provider practices that are inconsistent with sound fiscal, business, or medical practices, and result in an unnecessary cost to the Insurance provider or in reimbursement for services that are not medically necessary or that fail to meet professionally recognized standards for health care."

In 2011, $2.27 trillion was spent on health care and more than four billion health insurance claims were processed in the United States. It is an undisputed reality that some of these health insurance claims are fraudulent. No institution has undone more quickly and more completely than American medicine. In only a few decades, the medical system has been overrun by organizations seeking to exploit for profit the trust that susceptible and sick Americans place in their healthcare. Our legislators have proven themselves either unwilling or incapable of reining in the increasingly outrageous costs faced by patients, and market-based solutions only seem to funnel larger and larger sums of our money into the hands of corporations. Impossibly high insurance premiums and inexplicably large bills have become facts of life

Although health care fraud has many cons, they can be broken down into three major categories: 1. Phantom Billing. In this scenario, the provider bills Medicare for procedures, which are either unnecessary or not performed at all. Durable medical equipment false billings fall into this category as well. An example would be billing Medicare for a wheelchair or home care hospital bed which is either unneeded or undelivered.

2. False patient billing is often carried out in areas with large numbers of senior citizens, such as Florida, and the patient may be

duplicitous. For instance, for a kickback, a Medicare-eligible patient may provide his Medicare number and allow a provider to bill Medicare for tests and procedure either unneeded or unfulfilled.

3. Up coding and up billing seek to receive additional and unwarranted and illegal Medicare funds by using a code that may not be merited but results in the need for further services and tests, and, therefore, higher reimbursements. Billing for more expensive services or procedures than were actually provided or performed, commonly known as "upcoding" i.e., falsely billing for a higher-priced treatment than was actually provided (which often requires the accompanying "inflation" of the patient's diagnosis code to a more serious condition consistent with the false procedure code).

The majority of health care frauds are committed by a very small minority of dishonest health care providers. Unfortunately, the stock in trade of fraud-doers is to take advantage of the confidence that has been entrusted to them in order to commit ongoing fraud on a very broad scale.

Doctors have been caught performing medically unnecessary services solely for the purpose of generating insurance payments are seen very often in nerve-conduction and other diagnostic-testing schemes. They also misrepresent non-covered treatments as medically necessary covered treatments for purposes of obtaining insurance payments are widely seen in cosmetic-surgery schemes, in which non-covered cosmetic procedures such as "nose jobs" are billed to patients' insurers as deviated-septum repairs. Falsifying a patient's diagnosis to justify tests, surgeries or other procedures that aren't medically necessary constitutes fraud.

Unbundling which means billing each step of a procedure as if it were a separate procedure occurs as well. Billing a patient more than the co-pay amount for services that were prepaid or paid in full by the benefit plan under the terms of a managed care contract occurs as well. Accepting kickbacks for patient referrals is not uncommon.

Waiving patient co-pays or deductibles for medical or dental care and over-billing the insurance carrier or benefit plan (insurers often set the policy with regard to the waiver of co-pays through its provider contracting process; while, under Medicare, routinely waiving co-pays is prohibited and may only be waived due to "financial hardship").

Health fraud involves: selling drugs, devices, foods, or cosmetics that have not been proven effective, Wrongful or criminal deception intended to result in financial or personal gain, Submitting false bills or claims for service, or Falsifying medical records or medical reports is also against the rules.

Lying about credentials or qualifications, unnecessary medical treatment or drug prescriptions are other fraudulent examples. Health fraud scams can be found everywhere, promising help for many common health issues, including weight loss, memory loss, sexual performance, and joint pain. They target people with serious conditions like cancer, diabetes, heart disease, HIV/AIDS, arthritis, Alzheimer's, and many more. Health care fraud is a type of white-collar crime that involves the filing of dishonest health care claims in order to turn a profit.

Medical practitioner schemes include: individuals obtaining subsidized or fully-covered prescription pills that are actually unneeded and then selling them on the black market for a profit; billing by practitioners for care that they never rendered; filing duplicate claims for the same service rendered; altering the dates, description of services, or identities of members or providers; billing for a non-covered service as a covered service; modifying medical records; intentional incorrect reporting of diagnoses or procedures to maximize payment; use of unlicensed staff; accepting or giving kickbacks for member referrals; waiving member co-pays; and prescribing additional or unnecessary treatment.

Members can commit health care fraud by providing false information when applying for programs or services, forging or selling prescription drugs, using transportation benefits for non-medical related purposes, and loaning or using another's insurance card.

According to the Food and Drug Administration (FDA), a health product is fraudulent if it is deceptively promoted as being effective for a disease or health condition but has not been scientifically proven safe and effective for that purpose. A successful prosecution of a health care provider who ends in a conviction can have serious consequences. The health care provider faces incarceration, fines, and possibly losing the right to practice in the medical industry. Health care fraud remains a serious problem for these programs.

The U.S. Government Accountability Office has designated Medicaid as a program that is at high risk for improper payments.

Inappropriate payments "include those made for treatments or services that were not covered by program rules, that were not medically necessary, or that were billed for but never provided." There are a number of Federal and State laws to deter and punish those who fraudulently seek to obtain improper payments from Medicaid.

The False Claims Act establishes civil liability for offenses related to certain acts, including knowingly presenting a deceitful or fraudulent claim to the government for payment, and making a false record or statement that is material to the false or fraudulent claim. In June, 2002, for example, a Chicago cardiologist was sentenced to 12-1/2 years in federal prison and was ordered to pay $16.5 million in fines and restitution after pleading guilty to doing 750 medically unnecessary heart catheterizations, along with unneeded angioplasties and other tests as part of a 10-year fraud scheme.

The Anti-Kickback Statute, found in Section 1128B (b) of the Social Security Act, prohibits the knowing and willful offer, payment, solicitation, or receipt of any remuneration, in cash or in kind, to induce or in return for referring an individual for the furnishing or arranging of any item or service for which payment may be made under a Federal health care program. Remuneration means anything of value and can include gifts, under-market rent, or payments that are above fair market value for the services provided.

When a person's name or other identifying information is used without that person's knowledge or consent to obtain medicinal services or goods, or to submit false insurance claims for payment, that's medical identity theft. Medical identity theft frequently results in erroneous information being added to a person's medical record, or even the creation of an entirely fictitious medical record in the victim's name. According to the health trade publication HIPAA Journal, more hospitals and doctors' practices reported breaches in 2016 than in any other year since the U.S. Department of Health and Human Services' Office of Civil Rights, which collects data on leaks, started publishing breach summaries in 2009.

Among the latest leaks: Bronx-Lebanon Hospital Center in New York City left patients' names, home addresses, medical and mental health diagnoses, addiction histories, HIV statuses and even sexual assault and domestic violence reports exposed online because of a misconfigured backup server that stored the medical data.

Two years ago, Anthem Inc. notified 80 million customers that their personal health information may have been stolen after the insurer was hit by a sophisticated cyber-attack.

Other illegal medical activities include billing for services that were not actually performed. Billing for services that were performed by another provider. Billing for non-covered, services using an incorrect diagnosis code in order to have services covered, Billing a patient more than the co-pay amount for services provided for under the health insurance plan. And waiving patient co-pays or deductibles and over-billing the insurance plan. Waiving a copayment entices patients to get free services that may not be needed to enrich the medical provider.

Hospital systems, which are managed by business executives, behave like predatory lenders, pursuing patients and seizing their homes. Research charities are in bed with big pharmaceutical companies, which covertly profit from the donations made by working people. Patients receive bills in code, from entrepreneurial doctors they never even saw.

If patients complain, they discover that no one seems to care, or that no one has the resources to do anything about it. The managed care environment produces scams involving underutilization, and the withholding of medical care schemes that are harder to uncover and investigate, and much more dangerous to human health.

There is however, a remedy for this problem and is called the 'Whistleblower program'. With this program individuals can receive payments from the Government for reporting health care fraud. This book addresses the types of fraud which plague the healthcare industry and describes the most common fraudulent behavior throughout this industry and how to report fraud and possibly receive a reward. It is recommended that a person use an attorney to help file the Whistleblower claim.

If you properly report Medicare fraud, you may be entitled to a significant whistleblower reward. Fighting Medicare fraud is an important part of safeguarding our healthcare for future generations. Because Medicare is paid for almost exclusively by tax revenue, fraud hurts everyone. If you suspect that something has happened illegally, then it is your duty to blow the whistle. Doing so makes you part of the solution.

2. Health Care Fraud is a Crime

Medicare fraud and healthcare fraud in general is illegal. The US Office of Management and Budget says, "Improper payments" made by Medicare in 2010 amounted to more than $47.8 billion. That represents almost 10% of the $528 billion total Medicare spend that year. Fraud, waste, and abuse pose major risks for the healthcare system. Fraud means an intentional deception or misrepresentation made by a person with the knowledge that the deception could result in some unauthorized benefit to himself or some other person." "Abuse means provider practices that are inconsistent with sound fiscal, business, or medical practices, and result in an unnecessary cost to the Insurance provider or in reimbursement for services that are not medically necessary or that fail to meet professionally recognized standards for health care."

Although health care fraud has many cons, it can be broken down into three major categories: 1. Phantom Billing. In this scenario, the provider bills Medicare for procedures, which are either unnecessary or not performed at all. Durable medical equipment false billings fall into this category as well. An example would be billing Medicare for a wheelchair or home care hospital bed which is either unneeded or undelivered.

2. False patient billing is often carried out in areas with large numbers of senior citizens, such as Florida, and the patient may be duplicitous. For instance, for a kickback, a Medicare-eligible patient may provide his Medicare number and allow a provider to bill Medicare for tests and procedure either unneeded or unfulfilled. Up coding and up billing seek to receive additional and unwarranted and illegal Medicare funds by using a code that may not be merited but results in the need for further services and tests, and, therefore, higher reimbursements.

Providers who engage in fraud and abuse are subject to sanctions under a number of Federal and State laws. Sanctions under Federal law, for example, can take the form of administrative, civil, and criminal penalties. These penalties range from monetary fines and damages to prison time and exclusion from the Federal healthcare programs. Becoming familiar with common types of fraud, waste, and abuse, will better position providers to ensure they or their patients are not involved in such conduct. Although the following examples involve violation of Federal laws, many states have similar laws against fraud, waste, and abuse.

3. Medical Identity Theft involves the misuse of a person's medical identity to wrongfully obtain health care goods, services, or funds. Medical identity theft has been defined as "the appropriation or misuse of a patient's or a provider's unique medical identifying information to obtain or bill public or private payers for fraudulent medical goods or services."

Medical identity theft refers to the misuse of another individual's identifying medical information to receive medical care. Beyond the financial burden on patients, hospitals, health insurance companies, and government insurance programs, undetected cases pose major patient safety challenges. Inaccuracies in the medical record may persist even after the theft has been identified because of restrictions imposed by patient privacy laws. Be aware that stolen physician identifiers can be used to fill fraudulent prescriptions, refer patients for unnecessary additional services or supplies, or bill for services that were never provided.

Some people use the beneficiary medical identifiers to fraudulently bill services or items not provided, or to enable an ineligible person to receive services by impersonating a beneficiary. Billing for Unnecessary Services or Items by physicians also occurs. Providers are responsible for ensuring authorized services meet the definition of medical necessity in the States where they practice. To be covered by insurance the billed service or supply must be provided.

Some providers bill Medicaid for a covered service or item but do not deliver the service or item. These providers may create false records in an attempt to justify the bills. For example, a physician might sign charts and submit bills for examinations and tests that never took place. Providers should only bill for the medically necessary or otherwise authorized services or items provided to the beneficiaries.

Up coding is a term that is generally understood as billing for services at a higher level of complexity than the service actually provided. For example, a pain physician might bill for a steroid injection with X ray, but no X-ray machine was ever used. The physician payment is more when the procedure is done with an X-ray machine.

Unbundling is the practice of submitting bills in a fragmented fashion in order to maximize the reimbursement for various tests or procedures that are required to be billed together at a reduced cost. For example, a physician may order a urine drug screen panel which tests for many substances in a patient's urine to ascertain patient compliance. Instead of billing for the whole panel, the laboratory might attempt to increase income by billing for each test separately.

Kickbacks can be defined as offering, soliciting, paying, or receiving remuneration to induce, or in return for referral of patients or the generation of business involving any item or service for which payment may be made under Federal health care programs. For example, it would be illegal for a physician to accept payments from a medical imaging facility for referring patients.

A patient should learn some of the basic health care provider schemes and how to deter them from taking some easy money such as: billing for services not rendered, Billing for a non-covered service as a covered, service misrepresenting dates of service, Misrepresenting locations of service, Misrepresenting provider of service, Waiving of deductibles and/or co-payments, Incorrect reporting of diagnoses or procedures, Overutilization of services, Corruption (kickbacks and bribery), False or unnecessary issuance of prescription drugs. Billings for services and care not rendered are not uncommon. Providers might make more money by reporting they visited with or and treated the same patient on two separate days rather than one day. Each office visit is usually considered a different billable service.

It is not uncommon that somebody may impersonate a physician and bill for treatment. Medical doctors sign insurance claim forms showing that they had provided care but in reality, lesser-educated health professionals actually conducted the treatment. Most government health care plans and insurance companies don't allow medical providers or facilities to waive patients' deductibles or co-payments. The rationale may be that if patients have to pay something to see doctors, they'll only seek care if they really need it.

Regardless, some providers do waive patients' deductibles or co-payments and then submit other false claims to insurance companies to make up the dollar difference. Truly unscrupulous providers also will add a bunch of other deceitful services to the claim forms to increase their illegal gains knowing that the patients are unlikely to complain because their co-payments and deductibles were waived.

Listing an incorrect diagnosis or procedure is fraudulent. Unscrupulous providers can bill for extra services if they report procedures performed. Like all industries, the potential for corruption in the health care industry is great. Providers have been known to unlawfully pay for and/or receive payment for referrals. Obviously, that practice can lend itself to abuse when referrals are made for services that aren't even needed, such as X-rays, MRIs, prescription drugs, etc.

Prescription-drug abuse is sometimes defined as taking prescription medication for reasons beyond physicians' intentions. Pain killers are the most commonly abused prescription. These drugs' street value is almost 10 times the legal prescription value. Media around the country often report that thieves have robbed pharmacies at gunpoint to get painkillers. Crime prevention tips often suggest that homeowners should ensure that individuals don't have unneeded access to the occupants' prescription drugs.

Some patients doctor shop to obtain drug prescriptions. The doctors usually have no idea that the patients have already visited other physicians to obtain the same or other drugs. Impostors can easily recover the cost of the doctors' visits and filling of prescriptions by selling some or all the drugs on the street. Some patients and medical facility employees have taken prescription paper pads and forged prescriptions and provider signatures on them. Others make pen-and-ink changes to the quantity and/or authorized refill numbers on the paper prescriptions. (Electronic prescriptions from providers to pharmacists are helping prevent this fraud.)

A pharmacist previously stole large quantities of painkillers from his employer's inventory and then electronically submitted false claims to insurance companies using names of other beneficiaries' and their insurance policy numbers, which he obtained from his employer's computer. A pharmacist could also alter the quantity listed on legitimately received prescriptions for drugs, and manipulate the patients' paperwork and receipts or make co-payments like the above pharmacist and steal the extra drugs for himself.

Joint investigation by the FBI, DEA, U.S. Department of Health and Human Services-Office of Inspector General and Blue Cross Blue Shield of Michigan revealed that patients were getting prescriptions for narcotics for no medical purpose from a pain management clinic. Patients were recruited to come into the office and agree to diagnostic tests. In return, they would receive cash or prescriptions for Vicodin,

OxyContin, or Opana ER. Some patients agreed to get prescriptions for narcotics and then immediately turn them over to a recruiter. The recruiters were filling the prescriptions for resale on the streets.

In a typical visit, a patient would agree to medical tests such as blood tests, breathing tests, EKGs, EEGs, ultrasounds, X-rays, and psychological testing, no matter what their supposed medical problems were. The testing was all done before being seen by the doctor. All these tests were being billed to Blue Cross Blue Shield of Michigan and Medicare. The investigation revealed that for some of the tests that the clinic billed, the equipment was broken or the clinic did not even own the necessary equipment.

In addition to the prescription of narcotics, a large part of the practice conducted at the clinics was to provide patients with injections of lidocaine combined with steroids, which at times provided temporary relief of various joint and muscle pain. Although the injections given to the patients were superficial, they were billed falsely to the insurance companies as facet joint injections, paravertebral injections, sacroiliac nerve injections, sciatic nerve injections, and various nerve block injections.

Low back pain (LBP) has a major economic impact in the United States, with total costs related to this condition exceeding $100 billion per year. In the United States, patients with musculoskeletal conditions incur total annual medical care costs of approximately $240 billion. The reasons for long-lasting pain are many, from cancer and multiple sclerosis to back pain and arthritis. Adults with low back pain are often in worse physical and mental health than people who do not have low back pain. A study cited by WebMD, the average estimated annual medical expenditures for adults with back pain in 2005 was $6,096, while the estimated annual medical expenditure for those without pain was $3,516. Treating spine problems in the United States cost $85.9 billion a year, while cancer treatment, which costs $89 billion.

One doctor in Texas served prison time for health-care fraud. An-other has been disciplined by regulators five times, on charges, including dangerous overuse of anesthesia. A third devotes his practice to a controversial therapy that Medicare won't cover. Researchers have found that up to 42 percent of Medicare patients experience unnecessary treatment. Is this criminal behavior? White-collar crimes are characterized by "deceit, concealment, or violation of trust and are not dependent on the application or threat of physical force or violence. Health care fraud is a form of white-collar crime that may be committed by health care providers, consumers, companies providing medical supplies or services, and health care organizations.

The FBI has functioned as the primary investigative agency for health care fraud in both the public and private health systems. The Financial Crimes Section of the FBI was created in the 1980s. It comprises three units, one of which is devoted to health care fraud. The FBI has developed several national initiatives, including the Internet Pharmacy Fraud Initiative, the Auto Accident Insurance Fraud Initiative, and the Outpatient Surgery Center Initiative. The FBI has emphasized the investigation of medical professionals who engage in schemes that can directly harm patients. Such schemes include performing unnecessary surgeries, diluting medication for profit, and inappropriate prescribing practices.

The FBI previously announced indictments against 53 persons in Detroit, and Miami accused of conspiring to submit more than $50 million in false Medicare claims. It was alleged that at least nine Medicare provider companies as well as company executives, doctors, therapists, medical recruiters, medical assistants, and Medicare consumers participated in these schemes, which involved billing for physical therapy, occupational therapy, and infusion therapy that had not been provided.

Law enforcement is beginning to use technology to monitor discrepancies in billing as a means of preventing and identifying health care fraud. The Medicaid Anti-Kickback Statute prohibits knowingly and willfully paying or receiving any remuneration directly or indirectly, overtly or covertly, in cash or in kind in exchange for or to induce referrals of program-related business, including prescribing, purchasing, or recommending any service, treatment, or item for which payment will be made by Medicare, Medicaid, or any other federally funded health care program.

Physicians may perform unnecessary procedures to increase reimbursement, which may compromise patient safety. When medical providers bill for services never rendered, they create a false medical history for patients that may later cause them difficulty in obtaining disability or life insurance policies. When physicians bill the government for medical services that are not needed by the patient, they violate the trust placed in them by their patients and the government to provide only medically necessary care. The FDA describes health fraud as "articles of unproven effectiveness that are promoted to improve health, well-being or appearance." The articles can be drugs, devices, foods, or cosmetics for human or animal use.

Health care consumers need to identify these health care fraudsters and report them to attempt to salvage the health care system. People need to remember that he/she could receive a monetary reward for being a whistle blower.

As stated in the previous chapter, there are people who expose unethical or illegal wrongdoing within companies by reporting it internally to superiors or externally to the media, government authorities, or specialized attorneys. They can be either current or past employees (insiders), or outside individuals who are familiar with the unlawful conduct, and are not required to be U.S. citizens. If you properly report Medicare fraud, you may be entitled to a significant whistleblower reward.

Patients must be aware that there are aggressive physicians and conservative physicians. A patient should not have a treatment done unless it is medically necessary. When in doubt about a particular medical treatment it is prudent to get a second opinion from another doctor.

3. Whistleblowers

Whistle blowers are people who expose unethical or illegal wrongdoing within companies by reporting it internally to superiors or externally to the media, government authorities, or specialized attorneys. They can be either current or past employees (insiders), or outside individuals who are familiar with the unlawful conduct, and are not required to be U.S. citizens. If you properly report Medicare fraud, you may be entitled to a significant whistleblower reward.

The majority of successful whistle blower cases that are brought under the False Claims Act (FCA) involve healthcare fraud. Because millions of Americans are insured with federal or state government funds, healthcare is an area ripe for fraud. Medicare, Medicaid, and Tri-Care Veterans' benefits pay money for the care of individuals. Government employees also have their healthcare paid for with government funds.

Fraudulent claims involving government healthcare programs cost taxpayers billions of dollars each year and cause health care costs to rise. The False Claims Act is the government's central tool in identifying and prosecuting false claims for government funds under a variety of government contracts, including Medicare and Medicaid. While billions of dollars in healthcare fraud have been exposed through whistle blower reporting under the False Claims Act, it is estimated that billions of dollars in additional healthcare fraud remain undetected.

Healthcare fraud is the type of illegal industry that is worth billions of dollars. In fact, many men and women have made an estimate that around ninety billion dollars are lost to fake healthcare claims. Healthcare fraud is a scam that can hurt others. In addition, healthcare fraud can make other men and women pay higher insurance premiums. Co-payments and taxes are also affected.

If you believe that, you are able to report healthcare fraud you may want to follow a series of steps. First, you will need to gather information about the person you think is taking advantage of healthcare fraud. This means that you will need to obtain the name of the clinic that is involved with this healthcare fraud. You will also need to obtain the names of the doctors and the pharmacists who are a part of the healthcare fraud. You may want to contact a health fraud attorney to assist you in your claim. A Web search will give you names of attorney specialists near you.

After you have gathered the names of all the men and women who are involved you will need to make copies of documents that show examples of why you think that someone is faking healthcare problems. You should keep a diary of phone calls as well. This should include the dates, the times, and the people you spoke to on the phone. You should also state the outcome of the call. If you plan to report healthcare fraud, it is important for you to have as much information as possible.

Now you need to find out how you can contact the Insurance Fraud Bureau in your specific state. You can normally locate the Insurance Fraud Bureau in your state on the Coalition against Insurance Fraud Web site. However, you may need to contact your state's Department of Insurance if your state does not have an Insurance Fraud Bureau.

Once you go to either Web site, you will need to call the hot line number that is listed on the Web site. After contacting a representative, you will need to provide the representative with the name of the insurance agency that is being scammed. You will also need to provide any other information and details that you know of the healthcare fraud.

After you have contacted the Department of Insurance or the Insurance Fraud Bureau, you will need to contact the insurance company that the person is swindling. You can locate the insurance company's phone number on its Web site.

If you need to report Medicare fraud or Medicaid healthcare fraud, you will need to call your state's Department of Health and Human Services. If you cannot contact your state's Department of Health and Human Services, you will need to contact the Office of Inspector General Fraud.

You can normally contact the Inspector General or the Department of Health and Human Services by e-mail or by phone. You should provide information about the person who has committed the healthcare fraud, how it happened, or where it happened. Your identity will be protected. You can also contact the NICB through the e-mail, by calling, or by texting.

Several laws provide whistle blowers with financial rewards when they submit information that helps the government recover funds from companies or individuals committing fraud. Over the past 30 years, the U.S. authorities have paid hundreds of millions in total awards, with an average payout of approximately $1.5 million.

If you want to report an ongoing or widespread fraud you witnessed within your workplace, you need to be sure that you possess enough information to build a solid case. If you can back up your information with insider knowledge or substantial physical evidence, you may have a chance of becoming a successful whistle blower and take the first step. The whistle blower programs, laws, and several practical policies protect those who decide to come forward in several ways. Claims can be filed anonymously, and the relator is always shielded against all forms of retaliation since restitution, and reinstatement are always granted by the Government.

Several laws provide whistle blowers with financial rewards when they submit information that helps the government recover funds from companies or individuals committing fraud. Over the past 30 years, the U.S. authorities have paid hundreds of millions in total awards, with an average payout of approximately $1.5 million.

Laws have been passed to help protect whistle blowers from retaliation for reporting violations of the law, such as Medicare fraud. No longer can an employer be immune from liability for retaliation when an employee is engaged in protected activity. Corporations can no longer demand that its employees remain blindly loyal and silence them with threats. Nolan Auerbach views its clients as heroes for having the courage to step forward and become whistle blowers in healthcare fraud cases. Cases range from pharmaceutical fraud, medical device fraud, and hospital fraud, involving conduct from cost report violations, to kickbacks, to Stark violations.

Whistle blowers are usually long-time loyal employees who sit fairly high in the corporate organization and have a strong moral constitution. The primary motivation of the whistle blower is to correct wrongdoing. There is good news for whistle blowers or potential whistle blowers: If you work for a company or organization that you legitimately believe is defrauding the government, the law is on your side, particularly if your employer has retaliated against you.

The federal False Claims Act is specifically designed to encourage citizens to report fraud and to protect them from retaliatory actions; this protection also extends to a contractor or agent. If you or one of your family members is fired, demoted, suspended, threatened, or otherwise discriminated against because you tried to stop your employer from cheating the federal government, you have standing to sue.

Here are some things you need to know as a potential Whistle Blower:

1. You have to be able to prove that you made efforts to stop or correct improper actions that violate the False Claims Act. It is not required that you tell your employer that you are planning on filing a qui tam lawsuit. Title 31 U.S.C. Section 3730(h) prohibits retaliatory actions against any employee, contractor or agent who take lawful actions in furtherance of a False Claims Act. This anti-retaliation statute reflects the 2009 Congressional revisions to include both current and former employees, as well as contractors and agents. The types of retaliation action covered by the statute include discharge, demotion, suspension, threats, or harassment.

2. The protection of the retaliation statute applies if the whistle blower believes in good faith that his employer is violating the False Claims Act, whether or not they are correct in their belief. 31 U.S.C. 3730(h)(1) requires that the employee was engaged in protected activity, that he was retaliated against because of that activity, and that the whistle blower's employer knew he was engaged in protected activity. This protected activity also includes the process of investigating or determining whether or not fraud occurred. It is not required that an employer be told that a whistle blower has hired an attorney or intends to file a qui tam lawsuit. Rather, the employer can be sufficiently notified if a whistleblower tells his manager or supervisor that he is concerned about possible Medicare fraud, improper billing or raises concerns about off-label marketing or kickbacks.

3. You may be able to recover damages from your employer for the losses you have actually sustained. "Being made whole" addresses the kind of damages you may expect, like double your back pay, plus interest, if you have been fired. You also would be entitled to reinstatement with the same seniority. The False Claims Act anti-retaliation section specifically provides remedies under 31 U.S.C. Section 3730(h)(2) that are available to a whistle blower which include reinstatement with the same seniority status that the whistleblower would have had but for the discrimination, two times the amount of back pay, interest on the back pay, and compensation for any special

damages sustained as a result of the discrimination, including litigation costs and reasonable attorneys' fees.

4. You will not be entitled to "punitive" damages, but you may be entitled to compensation for pain and suffering as a result of any alleged emotional stress you have experienced.

5. Be sure that you have "reasonable" grounds for alleging that your employer is committing fraud. What is "reasonable"? If you have seen a pattern of falsified billing records, if you have proof that government entities are routinely billed for services or products they have not received, then you have "reasonable" indications that your employer is committing ongoing fraud. To prove fraud, you have to be able to demonstrate a pattern, a conscious attempt to deceive the government. Do not confuse your desire to "get even" with your ability to produce actual proof.

6. Act on proof, not suspicion. Do not let your emotions cause you to jump into a lawsuit because you do not like your supervisor, or you are otherwise unhappy with your workplace.

7. Seek professional advice immediately. Potential whistle blowers should consult a qualified attorney which can provide guidance about gathering evidence and navigating potential minefields. Just because you think there may be smoke in a given instance does not mean that there will be enough to light a legal fire. It is just as important for you to find out that you probably do not have a case as it is for you to learn that you do.

8. If you have grounds to file a whistle blower retaliation claim, you might also have grounds to file a False Claims Act or qui tam lawsuits based on your employer's submission of false claims to the federal government.

Fraudulent claims are among the most prevalent and serious business risks that insurance companies face. Many consumers have devised elaborate and clever schemes to benefit from defrauding their insurance providers, so insurance companies with the help of some government protection attract whistle blowers to fight back. Whistle blowers can even profit from the exposure of instances of insurance fraud.

Just as individuals have the right to help the government reclaim defrauded funds under the False Claim Act, consumers have the right to help insurance providers stop fraud through various hotlines, fraud bureaus and even the National Insurance Crime Bureau.

A whistle blower is most popularly thought of as someone who exposes political or corporate corruption, but there are also whistle blowers that help businesses escape from unethical consumer practices. The most common type of whistle blowing for insurance companies, by far, involves fraudulent insurance claims. In other words, one customer tries to game the system to make money, and another customer (the whistle blower) reported the unethical activity to the authorities.

There are other types of crimes that whistle blowers can aid insurance companies with, including violations of state or federal laws, company policies and codes of ethics, endangerment to the public safety or even internal corruption.

The specific procedure for whistle blowing depends on the type of scam, the agency or company being reported to, and the state where the suspicious activity is occurring. Most states have established bureaus for fraud detection. Most of these look for Medicaid and Medicare fraud, but private insurance fraud is normally reportable. If not, a whistle blower can contact the insurance company directly or call the local police. It's possible that the insurance company will reward a whistle blower for aiding in successful fraud avoidance.

Whistle blowers should present full details of the suspected scam, any important names or dates, phone numbers, addresses, and the amount of money believed to be targeted. The most common actions that lead to whistle blowing in medical billing are described below:

Up coding fraud: Upcoding fraud occurs when a healthcare provider submits a claim for healthcare services that represents a more serious and more expensive procedure than that which actually was performed.

Unbundling: Government healthcare programs often have special reimbursement rates for groups of procedures that are typically performed together. One common type of fraud is to "unbundled" these procedures or tests and bill each one separately, which results in greater reimbursement than the group reimbursement rate.

Lack of Medical Necessity: In order to qualify for payment by government healthcare programs, healthcare services, treatments, diagnostic tests, medical devices, and pharmaceuticals must be medically necessary. One common type of fraud is to submit claims for services, treatments, diagnostic tests, and medical devices that are not medically necessary.

False Certification: When healthcare providers submit bills to government healthcare programs. They are required to include certifications, including that the services were medically necessary, were actually performed, and were performed in accordance with all applicable rules and regulations. One common type of fraud involves falsifying these certifications in order to get a healthcare claim paid or to obtain additional business.

Inflating Overhead Cost: Medicare and other government healthcare programs reimburse hospitals and healthcare institutions for certain overhead and costs in addition to healthcare treatment. Hospitals are required to file Cost Reports with Medicare, providing information on the hospital's charges, revenue, profits, and charge-to-cost ratios, which determine how much Medicare will pay. One common type of fraud involves hospitals inflating the costs on their Medicare Cost Reports, or falsifying the information for these reports to maximize their Medicare reimbursement.

The Federal Anti-Kickback Statute and the Stark Laws both prohibit kickbacks to doctors and seek to prevent healthcare billing fraud. Any offer, payment, solicitation, or receipt of money to induce or reward the referral of patients or healthcare services is considered a kickback. These improper payments come in many different forms, including: referral fees; finder's fees; productivity bonuses; discounted leases; discounted equipment rentals; research grants; speaker's fees; excessive compensation; and free or discounted travel or entertainment. The offer, payment, solicitation, or receipt of any such monies or remuneration can be a violation of these laws.

The retail value of prescription drugs filled annually in the United States exceeds $300 billion per year. Spending on drugs through Medicare's Part D prescription-drug program totaled $103.7 billion in 2013, including spending by government, insurers and beneficiaries. The immense size and scope of the prescription-drug industry make it an appealing target for government fraud.

The Medicare prescription program, called Medicare Part D, began in 2006 and helps pay for most drugs sold through retail and mail-order pharmacies for roughly 36 million elderly and disabled Americans. Part D is structured differently than traditional Medicare: The federal government pays private companies to administer the benefit, and they in turn pay for the drugs that patients pick up at their pharmacies. According to a report by the Wall Street Journal, out of nearly 3,500 drugs, the top 100 by total cost represented nearly 60% of total Medicare Part D spending.

Brand-name drugs for more common conditions like acid reflux (Nexium) and asthma (Advair) represented some of the largest drug expenditures, and drugs that are ripe for Medicare fraud and abuse. Because of the significant sums of government money available and the number of participants in the program, sometimes Part D plan sponsors and/or their Pharmacy Benefit Managers (PBMs) engage in fraudulent practices that result in the improper claims for payment to federal programs, and can therefore form the basis for claims under the False Claims Act.

Common pharmacy fraud schemes include: Prescription drug switching substituting a more expensive drug for a cheaper one, Billing for a false or nonexistent prescription, Billing multiple payers for the same prescription, Billing for brand-name drugs when generic drugs are dispensed, Filling less than the prescribed quantity of a drug,

In the pharmaceutical industry, whistle blower actions typically arise through the illegal manufacture, promotion, and sale of drugs that are subsidized or reimbursed by the government through federally funded healthcare programs such as Medicare, Medicaid, or Tricare.

The most common pharmaceutical fraud cases involve: Adulterating drugs or deliberately avoiding manufacturing regulations; the safety and efficacy of drugs to federal regulators; Promoting drugs for uses that the Food and Drug Administration has not approved; Providing financial incentives to doctors to prescribe certain drugs; and Overcharging federal healthcare programs for drugs.

Pharmaceutical whistle blowers can work for the government to stop the illegal activity and receive a reward by filing a "quit am" tam" lawsuit under the False Claims Act.

Under the False Claims Act, whistle blowers who file a quit am lawsuit to prosecute healthcare fraud are protected from whistle blower retaliation and job discrimination, and are eligible to receive up to 30% of the money recovered by the government if the lawsuit is successful. Between 2009 and 2015, the DOJ recovered $26.4 billion, with the bulk coming out of healthcare cases. In 2015 alone, the federal government recovered $3.5 billion in settlements and judgments from civil cases filed under the False Claims Act, and $1.9 billion came from cases related to the healthcare industry.

Some examples of the largest healthcare fraud settlements and whistle blower rewards received from cases filed under the Qui Tam Act includes:

Johnson & Johnson – Pharmaceutical

Settlement: $2.2 billion "to resolve criminal and civil liability arising from allegations relating to the prescription drugs Risperdal, Invega and Natrecor, including promotion for uses not approved as safe and effective by the Food and Drug Administration and payment of kickbacks to physicians and to the nation's largest long-term care pharmacy provider." It's one of the greatest health care fraud settlements in U.S. history, according to the Department of Justice. Whistle blower reward: $167.7 million divided among whistle blowers in Pennsylvania ($112 million), Massachusetts ($27.7 million) and California ($28 million).

Novartis – Pharmaceutical

Settlement: $370 million to settle claims that it gave kickbacks to specialty pharmacies in exchange for recommending two of its drugs, Exjade and Myfortic. Whistle blower reward: $66.4 million awarded to a former Novartis sales manager.

Amedisys Inc. – Nursing and Therapy Services

Settlement: $150 million "to the federal government to resolve allegations that from 2008 to 2010. they billed Medicare for nursing and therapy services that were medically unnecessary or provided to patients who were not homebound, and otherwise misrepresented patients' conditions to increase payments," according to the Department of Justice. Whistle blower reward: $26 million split collectively among former Amedisys employees.

Omnicare Inc. – Nursing Facility

Settlement: $124.4 million for allegedly offering improper financial incentives to nursing facilities in return for their continued patronage of Omnicare to supply drugs to elderly Medicare and Medicaid patients. Whistleblower reward: $17.24 million awarded to Donald Gale, a former Omnicare employee.

Adventist Health System – Hospital System

Settlement: $115 million to settle allegations that it improperly compensated physicians for referring patients to its facility and miscode claims sent to Medicaid and Medicare for reimbursement of physician services. Whistle blower reward: The amount of the whistle blowers'' rewards in this case has not been released.

4. Health Provider Fraud

Several surveys have revealed that doctors have a negative view of the Affordable Health Care Act and its impact on the practice of medicine. Here are five ways Obamacare harmed doctors: It added more patients to Medicaid. Beginning in 2014, Obamacare put an additional 19.6 million Americans into Medicaid. On average, Medicaid physician payments are only 56 percent of what private insurance pays.

Lower payment rates already discourage doctors from accepting Medicaid beneficiaries, which has led to access issues and hospital emergency room overcrowding. As more patients enroll in this broken program, it will place even more financial strain on physicians who treat them. Doctors will be faced with the decision to either discontinue treating Medicaid patients or accept even more patients at the lower payment rate.

Every year, doctor payments face the threat of deep cuts due to the Sustainable Growth Rate formula, which governs the growth of Medicare physician payments from year to year. However, it's well known that such drastic provider payment cuts would harm seniors' access to care, and Congress has passed a last minute "doc fix" each year since 2003 to avoid this. Still, an estimated payment reduction of 27 percent is scheduled to go into effect next year unless Congress passes another doc fix, which will cost an estimated $208 billion. This problem faces doctors and Congress every year, and Obamacare does nothing to solve it.

The average state, for every dollar that a private insurer pays a primary care physician to care for a patient, Medicaid pays 52 cents." Many states pay even less. New York, for example, pays 29 cents. Many poor patients who will be driven onto Medicaid by Obamacare will be unable to access care.

Obamacare uses the Independent Payment Advisory Board (IPAB), a board of 15 unelected bureaucrats, to contain cost growth in Medicare by finding ways to cut spending to meet a new budget target. The board is limited in how it can achieve its goal, but one avenue definitely available is to further ratchet down provider payments. As IPAB cuts reimbursements, seniors will experience growing access problems as doctors discontinue seeing Medicare beneficiaries. If IPAB elects to limit seniors' access to certain treatments and services which is also within its abilities patient choice and physician autonomy will also be sacrificed.

It exacerbates future physician shortage. America is projected to face a shortage of 91,500 doctors in 2020. Meanwhile, many surveys have concluded that American doctors have a negative view of Obamacare and its impact on the medical field. One survey found that Obamacare is motivating 43 percent of doctors to move up their retirement within the next five years. This will intensify the already existing doctor shortage.

Obamacare's massive amount of red tape and regulations will tear apart the doctor-patient relationship. Doctors will have to focus increasingly on government rules rather than the specific needs of their patients. Obamacare's increase of government coverage will make physicians increasingly dependent on unreliable government reimbursement for medical services. In addition, Obamacare links payment for providers to adherence to government measurements of care. A recent doctor survey found that 67 percent of doctors surveyed said Obamacare would not improve the doctor-patient relationship.

No class of American professionals have been more negatively impacted by Obamacare than physicians. Obamacare regulations, especially the requirement that most Americans have health insurance or pay federal fines is expected to create prime opportunities for illegal scammers and legal products that consumers mistakenly confuse for legitimate health insurance. For an upfront enrollment fee plus a paid monthly subscription, consumers supposedly get deep discounts on medical services from doctors, hospitals and dentists within the companies' networks.

In reality, the discounts are often no more favorable than those that individual uninsured patients could negotiate on their own. On its website, the Federal Trade Commission says that while some discount medical plans provide real discounts, others take people's money and offer very little in return. Obamacare unleashed a movement of illegal scams. The Federal Trade Commission and Better Business Bureau recently posted notices warning consumers about the possibility of identity theft due to the new health care law.

The Affordable Care Act requires every new health insurance plans to cover ten essential benefits, which are: ambulatory or outpatient care, emergency-room care, hospital treatments, lab testing, maternity care, mental health care, pediatric services, prescription drugs, preventive care, and rehabilitative care and equipment.

The Affordable Care Act has resulted in increases in medical services. Patients under this health plan receive many unneeded services. Health care providers in some situations now do unnecessary surgical procedures, order unnecessary laboratory studies, X rays, physical therapies and hospital admissions. The incidence of kickbacks to physicians has increased with as a result of Obama Care from pharmaceutical companies, surgical equipment companies, hospitals etc.

A multitude of working physicians are currently being disciplined by their respective state medical boards for findings that patients may want to know about things such as sexual misconduct, their own addiction problems, overprescribing controlled substances, and all sorts of other documented examples of unprofessional or dangerous doctoring. Though the odds are quite good that your doctor isn't one of them, it's important to know for sure.

Consumers must learn some of the basic health care provider schemes and how to deter them from taking some easy money. A former physician may be best remembered for masterminding a record $373 million home-health fraud scheme against Medicare and Medicaid using fake patients including some of homeless patients promising them cash, food stamps and groceries. An Alabama doctor was arrested for Medicaid Fraud and a long list of other crimes so that he could bill health care benefit programs for medically unnecessary tests and procedures.

A Detroit area doctor who authorities say gave cancer treatment drugs to patients who did not need it. This doctor gives chemo treatments to healthy patients. Two other doctors are accused of running a "pill mill" and selling prescriptions for drugs, including oxycodone and hydrocodone, to addicts and drug dealers, who would then sell the drugs on the streets.

In another situation, patients with Alzheimer's disease were sitting unsupervised inside a small room of a medical psychological care facility watching the movie "Forrest Gump" for the umpteenth time. Granted, it's a great movie, but each time the patients sat in front of the tube watching it; the facility submitted insurance claims for providing "group therapy."

Health care offenders inside and outside the industry include patients, payers, employers, vendors and suppliers, and providers, including pharmacists. Organized-crime crime rings and computer hackers also play roles in committing health care fraud. The difference between the health care realm and many other industries is its huge, alluring, easy pile of cash. Evidence that the medical provider or its facility submitted claim forms to government health care plans and/or insurance companies for services and care that were never provided and the corresponding patient files had no supporting documentation.

An allergy doctor was providing a treatment, which was considered experimental and therefore, not approved by government health care plans or other insurance companies. With a few strokes of a pen or taps on a keyboard, the allergy doctor submitted claim forms and still got paid for utilizing the experimental treatment. She accomplished this by calling it (and coding it) something else that was covered by insurance plans and policies.

Providers might make more money by reporting they visited with or and treated the same patient on two separate days rather than one day. Each "office visit" is usually considered a separate billable service. It's a chilling thought that somebody might impersonate a physician and bill for treatment, but it does happen. I've conducted numerous investigations in which medical doctors signed insurance claim forms showing that they had provided all the care but in reality, lesser-educated mental health professionals actually conducted the therapy.

Most government health care plans and insurance companies don't allow medical providers or facilities to waive patients' deductibles or co-payments. The rationale may be that if patients have to pay something to see doctors, they'll only seek care if they really need it. Perhaps it's also a way to offset some of the expenses. Regardless, some providers do waive patients' deductibles or co-payments and then submit other false claims to insurance companies to make up the dollar difference. Truly unscrupulous providers also will add a bunch of other false services to the claim forms to increase their illegal gains knowing that the patients are unlikely to complain because their co-payments and deductibles were waived.

Unscrupulous medical providers can bill for extra services if they report false serious diagnoses or procedures performed. For example, if an elderly patient reportedly fell inside a nursing home, a crooked provider could intentionally misdiagnose her with head trauma requiring the (unnecessary) use of a computed tomography (CT) scan and/or blood tests.

Unscrupulous providers use this scheme on hypochondriac patients. Tests and exams can go on indefinitely or at least as long as a patient still has coverage or can make payments. Alcohol and drug rehabilitation facilities are ripe for over utilization. Providers have been known to unlawfully pay for and/or receive payment for referrals. Obviously, that practice can lend itself to abuse when referrals are made for services that aren't even needed, such as X-rays, MRIs, prescription drugs, etc.

An oncologist forced poisonous chemotherapy drugs into patients for years, telling them they had cancer when they did not. He over-treated terminal cancer patients rather than letting them die peacefully. When he could profit from it, he also under-treated actual cancer patients. Six other physicians and a chiropractor have also been arrested for participating in a kickback scheme that netted them $200,000 worth of cash and gifts for referring 20,000 patients to a medical testing facility.

Health care consumers need to identify these health care fraudsters and report them to attempt to salvage the health care system. People need to remember that he/she could receive a monetary reward for being a whistle blower. Whistle blowers are people who expose unethical or illegal wrongdoing within companies by reporting it internally to superiors or externally to the media, government authorities, or specialized attorneys. They can be either current or past employees (insiders), or outside individuals who are familiar with the unlawful conduct, and are not required to be U.S. citizens. If you properly report Medicare fraud, you may be entitled to a significant whistleblower reward.

5. Hospital Fraud

Wikipedia defined a hospital as a health care institution providing patient treatment with specialized medical and nursing staff and medical equipment. A general hospital typically has an emergency department to treat urgent health problems ranging from fire and accident victims to a heart attack. A district hospital typically is the major health care facility in its region, with large numbers of beds for intensive care and additional beds for patients who need long-term care. Specialized hospitals include trauma centers, rehabilitation hospitals, children's hospitals, seniors' hospitals, and hospitals for dealing with specific medical needs such as psychiatric treatment (see psychiatric hospital) and certain disease categories. Specialized hospitals can help reduce health care costs compared to general hospitals.

A teaching hospital combines assistance to people with teaching to medical students and nurses. A medical facility smaller than a hospital is generally called a clinic. Hospitals have a range of departments (e.g.: surgery and urgent care) and specialist units such as cardiology. Some hospitals have outpatient departments, and some have chronic treatment units. Common support units include a pharmacy, pathology, and radiology.

Hospitals are usually funded by the public sector, by health organizations (for profit or nonprofit), by health insurance companies, or by charities, including direct charitable donations according to the National Health Care Anti-Fraud Association in the United States. If a patient is not scammed by a health care provider or a drug company, he/she may be scammed by a hospital instead. Hospitals are vulnerable to corruption. In the U.S., health care fraud has been estimated to cost $60 billion per annum, or 3% of total health care expenditures with much of it in the hospital sector. Hospitals account for 50% or more of health care spending in many countries. Fraud and corruption in hospitals negatively affect access and quality, as public servants make off with resources, which could have been used to reduce out of pocket expenditures for patients, or improve needed services.

In the broadest sense, Hospital Fraud can be broken down into three areas: 1. hospital inpatient fraud, 2. hospital outpatient fraud, and 3. cost report fraud. Within those broad areas, there are many ways in which a hospital system can run afoul of the False Claims Act, whistleblower cases exposing this system-wide fraud is increasing in numbers. Claims for inpatients must also avoid upcoding, unbundling of services, and contain duplicates.

With outpatient claims, the intentional manipulation of code assignments to maximize payments and avoid National Correct Coding Initiative (NCCI) edits constitutes fraud. The Outpatient Prospective Payment System (OPPS) rules require hospitals to submit claims for all OPPS services provided at the same hospital, to the same patient, on the same day, unless certain conditions are met. The submission of multiple claims for OPPS services delivered to the same patient on the same day may violate the False Claims Act. Hospitals are usually funded by the public sector, by health organizations (for profit or nonprofit), by health insurance companies, or by charities, including direct charitable donations according to the National Health Care Anti-Fraud Association in the United States.

There are common types of fraud, which occur in hospitals in low-income countries, and suggest ways to prevent and control fraud. Hospitals in low-income countries are particularly vulnerable to fraud in part because administrative systems are not well developed or transparent, making it hard to distinguish between intentional fraud, and abuse due to incompetence or ignorance. In addition, hierarchical structures and personnel management systems may discourage people from voicing concerns or pointing out poor performance for fear of retaliation.

A significant proportion of total False Claim Act violations, both in terms of the actual number of cases brought and in terms of dollars lost to fraud, waste, and abuse, occurs within the health care field, including fraud by hospitals and medical facilities. In 2010, hospitals and medical facilities were the targets of more than one-third of all civil fraud investigations. In today's world, health care is an enormous business, accounting for about $2.2 trillion in annual expenditures in the United States economy.

A landmark study published in 2000 by the Institute of Medicine of the National Academy of Sciences pointed out that up to 98,000 Americans may die in US hospitals annually due to preventable medical errors. These errors were classified as diagnostic, treatment-related, failure of preventative measures, communication issues, and other hospital system failures (JAMA, May 18, 2005; Commonwealth

Fund, May 27, 2005). The take-home message was that hospitals are large, cumbersome institutions with many moving parts operating in mutually exclusive fashion, frequently placing patients at risk for adverse events.

The types of improper behaviors that some hospitals may engage in include: Fraudulent coding of procedures, such as up coding or unbundling, paying kickbacks to physicians or other health care organizations in order to induce patient referrals Performing and billing for medically unnecessary procedures billing for services not actually performed, reporting higher than actual costs, entering into or having been existing financial relationships with health care providers who refer patients, Paying recruiters to deliver homeless Medicare or Medicaid beneficiaries by ambulance to the hospital for medically unnecessary treatments in order to bilk the government.

Fourteen hospitals around the country paid a total of $12 million to settle False Claims Act lawsuits alleging overcharges to Medicare from 2000 to 2008. The whistle blowers contended that the hospitals performed kyphoplasties, minimally-invasive spinal procedures, on an inpatient basis, rather than as an outpatient procedure, in order to obtain a higher reimbursement from Medicare. A medical center paid $22 million to resolve allegations that it violated the Federal Anti-Kickback Statute and the Stark Act.

The whistle blowers claimed that the hospital entered into eleven professional service agreements with a cardiology group by which the group received excessive payments. In exchange, the cardiology group referred cardiac procedures to the hospital over a ten-year period. The other whistle blower alleged that over an eight-year period, the hospital billed Medicare for out-patient cancer treatments not covered under Medicare or TRICARE by intentionally using incorrect procedure codes.

In the largest health care fraud case in history, hospital chain, HCA, agreed to pay the government $631 million to resolve allegations stemming from nine False Claims Act suits. It was alleged that HCA defrauded the government in numerous ways, including by inflating cost reports, billing for claims initiated by kickbacks to physicians for referrals, and billing for unallowable costs.

Federal officials have revealed the identity of a Fort Lauderdale orthopedic surgeon who blew the whistle on illegal physician kickbacks, complicit hospital administrators and negligent financial oversight at taxpayer-supported public hospital system to pay nearly $70 million to settle charges of healthcare fraud. Administrators awarded employment contracts to a group of top physicians, including cardiologists and other specialists, which paid the doctors more than fair market value based on their ability to increase patient referrals to the hospital system, in violation of federal law.

Even the simplest medical procedure can cost tens of thousands of dollars. One error could add several thousand dollars to an already hefty bill. Even if your insurance does cover the entire bill the excess cost will be passed along to you eventually in the form of higher insurance premiums so it's in everyone's best interest to detect and correct hospital billing errors.

If you've gone to the hospital to have your tonsils removed and see a reference to chemo-therapy it's going to stand out on the bill. Don't be afraid to make some phone calls to question this. You might have to pay for it yourself if your insurance refuses to pay it. Overcharges are one of the most common billing errors. Duplication is another common billing mistake. If you see the same charge listed more than once you should ask the hospital why. It may be a valid charge but this error is so common you shouldn't let it go unchallenged.

When you receive the billing from your hospital you should look to see if you were billed for services you never received. Did you get every service, treatment and medication for which you are being billed? Check your log carefully. If you find errors, contact your provider's billing office and your insurer. If they are of no help and the discrepancies are significant, you may want to turn to trained professionals who will help you analyze the bill and negotiate for you. You can also get help from the consumer protection office of your state's attorney general.

According to a Department of Justice announcement, two hospital groups which together run an acute-care hospital reportedly submitted false claims to Medicare and MediCal programs. The submitted claims improperly requested reimbursement for healthcare services rendered to patients referred by providers with whom the two companies had inappropriate financial relationships. A hospital administrator was convicted in March with two of his top executives of charges of paying hundreds of thousands of dollars in kickbacks to doctors for referring patients on Medicare or Medicaid to the struggling hospital.

Recently, 55 hospitals across 21 states agreed to pay more than $34 million combined to resolve resolving allegations that they billed Medicare for kyphoplasties on an inpatient basis rather than outpatient to inflate their Medicare reimbursements. With this latest settlement, the DOJ has now reached agreements with more than 100 hospitals totaling approximately $75 million to resolve allegations, they mischarged Medicare for kyphoplasties.

A hospital agreed to pay $4.9 million to resolve allegations that it over billed Medicare and Medicaid by keeping patients in its St. Joseph Medical Center in Towson, Md., longer than necessary. The hospital allegedly admitted and kept patients in the hospital for unnecessary "short stays," or one- to two-day admissions, from 2007 through 2009. Those allegedly unnecessary admissions were not tied to any one physician or department, which could have made them difficult to identify with an internal review.

A hospital created a for-profit entity to own four specialty limited liability companies that employed part-time physicians to perform outpatient surgeries and procedures at this hospital. This was done in response to competition from a nearby ambulatory surgical center, and the hospital allegedly paid the physicians improperly to discourage them from referring lucrative cases to competing facilities. The government may pursue enforcement with the anticipation that criminal actions against hospitals and health systems could result in their exclusion from federal healthcare programs, which could have significant repercussions if it is a major provider to the community.

This was evident in the recent case involving Raleigh, N.C.-based WakeMed Health & Hospitals. The case centered on allegations that WakeMed, an 870-bed system, billed Medicare for millions of dollars in overnight care when patients had actually received treatment and were released within the same day.

Chicago has been hit with a shocking corruption scandal involving taxpayer money. Federal authorities have raided a hospital on Chicago's West Side after alleged crimes of medically unnecessary sedation, intubation and tracheotomy procedures on patients in an attempt to defraud Medicare and Medicaid. The case also involves numerous questionable penile enlargement procedures, and a kickback scheme where doctors were paid by the hospital for making referrals to the hospital.

A former employee of a Mississippi hospital is getting almost $3.5 million as part of a string of settlements where 18 hospitals in seven states have agreed to pay $20.4 million over allegations, they broke federal law by receiving Medicare reimbursements for psychiatric services that were not "medically reasonable or necessary. The hospitals allegedly were aided by a patient recruiting operation on skid row that plucked homeless people from the streets and delivered them with fake medical conditions to the hospitals. They were receiving kickbacks up to $20,000 a month from some of these hospitals, and they were delivering between 30 and 50 patients a month.

The "patients" were picked up by recruiters who sent them to the center, where they were given a phony diagnosis, and forms were filled out justifying their eligibility for government medical programs. Medi-Cal and Medicare would be billed for the ambulance and hospital stay. After their hospital stays, the homeless patients would be returned to Skid Row shelters, but they would go back to the hospitals multiple times.

Federal prosecutors said several doctors at a Kentucky rural hospital performed procedures for unneeded coronary stents, pacemakers and diagnostic catheterizations, and then billed the federal programs. The doctors were affiliated with the clinic, a physician group that entered an exclusive arrangement with Saint Joseph in 2008 to provide cardiology services to the hospital's patients. Hospitals generally receive between $10,000 and $15,000 for medical procedures such as heart stents.

Hospitals and hospital systems may engage in improper or illegal behavior at the expense of taxpayers in order to gain a competitive edge in the health care marketplace or to obtain greater reimbursements from the federal government than they are entitled to receive. These organizations often are motivated by the fact of simple greed for more, and finer, profits.

The types of improper behaviors that some hospitals may engage in include: Fraudulent coding of procedures, such as up coding or unbundling, Paying kickbacks to physicians or other health care organizations in order to induce patient referrals, Performing and billing for medically unnecessary procedures, Billing for services not actually performed, Reporting higher than actual costs, Entering into or having existing financial relationships with health care providers who refer patients, Paying recruiters to deliver homeless Medicare or Medicaid beneficiaries by ambulance to the hospital for medically unnecessary treatments in order to bilk the government, Paying recruiters to deliver homeless Medicare or Medicaid beneficiaries by ambulance to the hospital for medically unnecessary treatments in order to bilk the government.

Fourteen hospitals around the country paid a total of $12 million to settle False Claims Act lawsuits alleging overcharges to Medicare from 2000 to 2008. The whistle blowers contended that the hospitals performed kyphoplasties, minimally-invasive spinal procedures, on an inpatient basis, rather than as an outpatient procedure, in order to obtain a higher reimbursement from Medicare. The two whistle blowers received $2.1 million as their share of the recovery.

A medical center paid $22 million to resolve allegations that it violated the Federal Anti-Kickback Statute and the Stark Act. The whistle blowers claimed that the hospital entered into eleven professional service agreements with a cardiology group by which the group received excessive payments. In exchange, the cardiology group referred cardiac procedures to the hospital over a ten-year period. The whistle blowers received nearly $3 million as their share of the recovery.

Hospitals are vulnerable to corruption. In the U.S., health care fraud has been estimated to cost $60 billion per annum or 3% of total health care expenditures and much of it is in the hospital sector. Hospitals account for 50% or more of health care pending in many countries. Fraud and corruption in hospitals negatively affect access and quality, as public servants make off with resources, which could have been used to reduce out-of-pocket expenditures for patients, or improve needed services.

A former employee of a Mississippi hospital is getting almost $3.5 million as part of a string of settlements where 18 hospitals in seven states have agreed to pay $20.4 million over allegations they broke federal law by receiving Medicare reimbursements for psychiatric services that were not "medically reasonable or necessary." Some nonprofit hospitals have engaged in the practice of charging inflated and inordinate rates for medical care to uninsured patients, while providing discounts to insured patients and those on Medicare or Medicaid. Also, the hospitals routinely utilize aggressive, abusive, and oppressive collection practices to recover this inflated medical debt. These practices include lawsuits filed against patients who are poor and indigent.

Over the years, some hospitals systems have become notorious for their practices resulting in fraud, waste, and abuse, and for their repeated violations of the False Claims Act. Hospitals and hospital systems may engage in improper or illegal behavior at the expense of taxpayers in order to gain a competitive edge in the health care marketplace or to obtain greater reimbursements from the federal government than they are entitled to receive.

More recently, federal officials arrested the owner and CEO of a hospital in Chicago, along with the hospital's CFO and several physicians. The case involved physicians allegedly receiving more than $225,000 in cash and other forms of payment for referring Medicare and Medicaid patients to the 119-bed hospital, as well as a federal inspection report that quoted some of the hospital staff recalling the provision of allegedly unnecessary tracheotomies on patients. The extraordinary evidence amassed by investigators along with the egregiousness of the allegedly unnecessary medical treatments and alleged threats to patient safety made this case criminal.

Whistle blowers are people who expose unethical or illegal wrongdoing within companies by reporting it internally to superiors or externally to the media, government authorities, or specialized attorneys. They can be either current or past employees (insiders), or outside individuals who are familiar with the unlawful conduct, and are not required to be U.S. citizens. If you properly report Medicare fraud, you may be entitled to a significant whistleblower reward.

6. Medical Necessity Fraud

Patients should attempt to ascertain if their medical treatment is actually medically necessary. Some physicians will fabricate a diagnosis so that a certain treatment is covered by a patient's health insurance. As expected, some physicians will fabricate a diagnosis so that the patient's insurance carrier will pay the provider. If the insurance denies the treatment, the patient will subsequently be responsible to pay the medical bill.

Medical necessity is a United States legal doctrine, related to activities which may be justified as reasonable, necessary, and/or appropriate, based on evidence-based clinical standards of care. In a small number of cases, Medicare may determine if a method of treating a patient should be covered on a case-by-case basis. Even if a service is medically determined to be "reasonable and necessary," coverage may be limited if the service is provided more frequently than allowed under Medicare coverage policies.

Understanding and determining medical necessity can be very complex for physicians, clinicians, coders, and billers. A physician or clinical provider of care may have a completely different understanding, interpretation, and definition of medical necessity than the patient or a patient's family member. A third-party insurance payer may also have another completely different understanding and application of the term.

Medicare and private payers recognize medical necessity as a deciding factor for claims payment. For more than thirty years public and private health insurance plans have used the term medical necessity as a place holder to define the limits of their benefit coverage, despite widespread disagreement about its meaning. Initially, medical necessity was used to ensure that providers were paid for services performed.

Medically Necessary" or "Medical Necessity" shall mean health care services that a Physician, exercising prudent clinical judgment, would provide to a patient for the purpose of evaluating, diagnosing or treating an illness, injury, disease or its symptoms, and that are: in accordance with the generally accepted standards of medical practice; clinically appropriate, in terms of type, frequency, extent, site and duration, and considered effective for the patient's illness, injury or disease; and not primarily for the convenience of the patient or Physician, or other Physician, and not more costly than an alternative service or sequence of services at least as likely to produce equivalent therapeutic or diagnostic results as to the diagnosis or treatment of that patient's illness, injury or disease.

Medical necessity refers to a decision by your health plan that your treatment, test, or procedure is necessary for your health or to treat a diagnosed medical problem. Most health plans will not pay for healthcare services that they deem to be not medically necessary. It's important to remember that what you or your doctor defines as medically necessary may not be consistent with your health plan's coverage rules. Before you have any procedure, especially one that is potentially expensive, review your benefit handbook to make sure it is covered. If you are not sure, call your health plan's customer service representative.

Health plans have appeals processes (made more robust under the Affordable Care Act) that allow patients and their doctors to appeal when a pre-authorization request is rejected. Medically necessary care (MNC) is the reasonable and essential diagnostic, preventive, and treatment services (including supplies, appliances, and devices) and follow-up care as determined by qualified health care providers, in treating any condition, disease, injury, or congenital or developmental malformation.

Medical necessity can also be confusing when it comes to who is going to pay for the procedure or services. Many third-party payers have specific coverage rules regarding what they consider medically necessary or have riders and exclusions for specific procedures. Third-party payers may have a specific exclusion for procedures that they consider experimental, unproven for a specific diagnosis, or cosmetic.

The Social Security Act's definition of medical necessity is all about payment and not necessarily about patient care. It's an important distinction, especially from compliance and coding perspective, and one that must be made clear in discussions with providers. Medical necessity is based on "evidence-based clinical standards of care". This means that there is evidence to support a course of treatment based on a set of symptoms or other diagnostic results.

Meeting medical necessity requirements is essential for the financial success of a medical office. The term "medical necessity" received a great deal of attention during the era of health care reform.

Each payer may have their own definition of medical necessity based on the above standard definition. These payers are any entity other than the patient that finances or reimburses a provider for medical services for a patient including; insurance carriers, third party payers, or medical sponsors such as a union or employer.

Physician must be thorough in their notes and explanations in order to give the payer's medical reviewers sufficient data from which to determine the necessity of a diagnosis, a set of tests, or a treatment or therapy. The medical transcription and medical records team must be equally as careful in their attention to detail in order to make sure all of the correct information is transmitted in a timely manner.

There are times when medical necessity is obvious, such as emergency situations. When a patient arrives at the emergency room by ambulance with chest pains, shortness of breath, and loss of consciousness, no one stops to consider whether the bill will be paid by the insurance carrier because the reasonable and customary course of treatment in this situation is to provide immediate, comprehensive health care services, to alleviate symptoms, and determine the reason for these symptoms.

Services or supplies that a Provider, exercising prudent clinical judgment, would provide to a patient for the purpose of preventing, evaluating, diagnosing or treating an illness, injury, disease or its symptoms, and that are: . In accordance with generally accepted standards of medical practice; . Clinically appropriate, in terms of type, frequency, extent, site and duration, and considered effective for the patient's illness, injury or disease. Even if a particular procedure or service is considered medically necessary, some payers impose limits on how many times a provider may render a specific service within a specified time frame.

Medical necessity documentation from a physician or provider should include the following: Severity of the "signs and symptoms" or direct diagnosis exhibited by the patient. This is our diagnosis driver, and multiple diagnoses may be involved. Probability of an adverse or a positive outcome for the patient, and how that risk equates to the diagnosis currently being evaluated. This is the medical risk vs. gain. Need and/or availability of diagnostic studies and/or therapeutic intervention(s) to evaluate and investigate a patient's presenting problem or current acute or chronic medical condition. In other words, does the facility, office, or hospital have what the provider or clinician needs to render care?

7. Pharmaceutical Company Fraud

Pharmaceutical company fraud has become the most common type of fraud pursued by the Federal government under the False Claims Act (FCA). Under the FCA, employees or citizens who have knowledge of fraudulent activities against the government can initiate a qui tam action to hold companies accountable for their illegal and fraudulent actions, and to reimburse the federal government. From 2007 through July 18, 2012, pharmaceutical companies paid over $17 billion in penalties to settle 67 federal cases brought by the U.S. Department of Justice. Of this amount, $14.48 billion (85%) of the penalties resulted from the settlement of qui tam lawsuits initiated by whistleblowers.

Some pharmaceutical companies conduct fraudulent clinical trials, making sure to bury any negative results that would show how dangerous their drugs really are. They buy the favor of the media by pumping hundreds of millions of dollars into magazine, television, newspaper and online advertising. According to criminal complaints, attorney general reports and other sources accused the specialty pharmaceutical company Insys Therapeutics with the help of several physicians across the country is putting profits before patient care as it makes millions off patients' pain syndromes. Insys is subject to investigations regarding the sales and marketing practices of its pain product Subsys Fentanyl, a painkiller delivered as an oral spray. The Scottsdale, Arizona-based Insys Therapeutics' company revenue is almost entirely derived from the highly addictive opiate fentanyl, which it markets under the brand-name Subsys Fentanyl.

In the six months which ended June 30, 2015, Subsys sales accounted for $147.2 million of $148.4 million in total revenue. The potency of Subsys also comes with a high price tag. One package of 30 sprays can cost between $900 and $3,000, depending on the dosage, and those prices only seem to be increasing. Subsys, according to FDA guidelines, is only meant to be used to treat late-stage cancer pain.

The suit alleges that the Company's management was aware that about 10% of prescriptions approved through the Prior Authorization Department were for cancer patients. The majority of prescriptions were written for peripheral neuropathy, lower-back pain and sciatica.

A sales representative admitted that she provided doctors with financial kickbacks in return for them overprescribing Insys. This drug is a controversial painkiller to insured patients, most of whom weren't approved for the drug under FDA guidelines. Furthermore, a connection could be more readily detected between the volume of Subsys prescriptions and payments to doctors.

Another unfortunate case involved Celebrex. The importance of Celebrex to Pfizer is indisputable. Officials made a strategic decision during the early trial to be less than forthcoming about the drug's safety. It is one of the company's best-selling drugs, racking up more than $2.5 billion in sales, and was prescribed to 2.4 million patients in the United States last year alone. Celebrex is still sold and heavily marketed, as if nothing would have happened. There is still no clinical proof that Celebrex is better at preventing serious gastrointestinal injuries. The truth was that Celebrex was no better at protecting the stomach from serious complications than other drugs.

A person must be aware that fake online pharmacies are scams that are designed to trick you into paying for items you will never receive, or items that do not live up to their claims. Scammers will set up fake pharmacy websites that are designed to look like legitimate retailers. They will offer health products, medicines and drugs at very cheap prices or without the need for a prescription from a doctor. Prescription-only medicine requires a doctor or other qualified healthcare professional to have examined you. Most medicines have at least some side-effects, and these can be very serious for some people. They can also have dangerous interactions with medicines you are already taking.

Be aware of some online fraudulent pharmacies. If you take up an offer, and pay the 'retailer', you may never receive the items you ordered. If you do receive the products that you order, there is no guarantee that they are the real thing. In some cases, the medicines or other products may even damage your health. But with the proliferation of counterfeit medicine, a growing number of Americans who use online pharmacies may be at risk for taking fake pills that can result in serious health problems or even death.

According to the Federal Drug Administration, drugs sold on bogus websites may contain the wrong ingredients, incorrect quantities of ingredients, or may be composed of materials like drywall and eggshells. Drugs like Viagra and painkillers were the prime focus for counterfeiters until the last 10 years or so, but now people are involved in faking a variety of drugs, including cancer drugs, blood pressure medicines and cholesterol medicines. According to the FDA, drugs like Ambien, Xanax, Lexapro, and Ativan are also being faked.

Among the sellers of opioids, none has been more successful or controversial than Purdue Pharma, the maker of the No. 1 drug in the class: OxyContin, which generated $3.1 billion in revenue in 2010. OxyContin's bad reputation, however, has obscured a significant step. Last year Purdue began selling a reformulated version that should help reduce the worst form of abuse. The original drug had a time-release mechanism that could be defeated by crushing the pill and snorting it, smoking it, or adding water to the powder and injecting it for a heroin-like high. Purdue's claims that the time-release process reduced the addiction risk were crucial in making doctors feel comfortable prescribing a powerful addictive drug.

By contrast, the new version of OxyContin breaks into chunks rather than a powder. If water is added, the result is the formation of a gelatinous mass. The drug wears off hours early in many people. OxyContin is a chemical counterpart of heroin, and when it doesn't last a 12-hour duration, patients can experience excruciating symptoms of withdrawal, including an intense craving for the drug. Over the last 20 years, more than 7 million Americans have abused OxyContin, according to the federal government's National Survey on Drug Use and Health. The drug is widely blamed for setting off the nation's prescription opioid epidemic, which has claimed more than 190,000 lives from overdoses involving OxyContin and other painkillers since 1999.

Doctors eventually discovered that the drug lasted around eight hours rather than 12, and that patients would crash, needing more and higher doses. Patients who took moderate amounts for backaches or arthritis could find themselves hooked. Addicts saw they could easily get high by crushing the pills and then snorting, chewing, or injecting them.

Mylan's EpiPen became the focus for scrutiny, as its price increased by nearly 500 percent over seven years. This device is potentially a life-saving device for allergies. The cost of the life-saving drug inside each EpiPen injector is worth a couple of dollars. When pharmaceutic companies face no competition in the market, pharmaceutic companies have the power to set whatever price they need, and patients then pay more for health insurance.

In another scenario, it's quite shocking that nearly three-quarters of all retracted drug studies are due to pure falsification of data. Especially when one considers that even well-researched drugs can still have significant side effects. Vioxx is perhaps one of the better examples of what can happen when a drug is manufactured and sold under false pretenses. It killed more than 60,000 people in just a few years' time, before it was removed from the market. In the case of Vioxx, there are lingering questions about the sound-ness of the original research used to back the drug initially. We are therefore confronted with indisputable evidence that the drug paradigm is about money, not health, and certainly not dependable scientific inquiry.

It's important to realize that all research is not published. It should therefore, come as no surprise that drug studies funded by a pharmaceutical company that reaches a negative conclusion will rarely be published. Drug companies spend far more on marketing drugs, which is almost twice as much than on developing drugs. Until recently, paying bribes to doctors to prescribe their drugs was commonplace at big pharmaceutical companies, although the practice is now generally frowned upon and is illegal in many places. GlaxoSmithKline (GSK) was fined $490m in China previously for bribery and has been accused of similar practices in Poland and the Middle East.

The rules on gifts, educational grants and sponsoring lectures, for example, are less clear cut, and these practices remain commonplace in the US. Furthermore, a previous study found that doctors in the US receiving payments from pharma companies were twice as likely to prescribe their drugs. This may well exacerbate the problem of overspending on drugs by governments.

For two years, federal prosecutors in at least four states have been working with the Defense Department and other agencies to investigate allegations that some of the firms, and their sales staff are committing healthcare and prescription fraud, selling expensive pain creams and other drugs not approved by the Food and Drug Administration to veterans and their families.

The use of compounded drugs by current and former servicemen and servicewomen has skyrocketed in the past decade; federal data show. They were paying illegal kickbacks to some doctors and medical professionals to issue prescriptions for compounded medications. Tricare officials say the beneficiaries are receiving calls or direct requests from sales representatives who ask whether patients have certain medical conditions, and if so, if they are interested in compound medications. They then ask the patients to complete forms and provide their sponsor's Social Security number to initiate the prescriptions while they bill Tricare. Such medications can range in cost from a few hundred dollars to more than $9,000 per prescription.

In the last few years, pharmaceutical companies have agreed to pay over $13 billion to resolve U.S. Department of Justice allegations of fraudulent marketing practices, including the promotion of medicines for uses that were not approved by the Food and Drug Administration. Pfizer was fined $2.3 billion, which was then the largest health care fraud settlement and the largest criminal fine ever imposed in the United States. Pfizer pled guilty to misbranding the painkiller Bextra with "the intent to defraud or mislead," promoting the drug to treat acute pain at dosages the FDA had previously deemed dangerously high. Bextra was pulled from the market in 2005 due to safety concerns.

Merck agreed to pay a fine of $950 million related to the illegal pro-motion of the painkiller Vioxx, which was withdrawn from the market in 2004 after studies found the drug increased the risk of heart attacks. The company pled guilty to have promoted Vioxx as a treatment for rheumatoid arthritis before it had been approved for that use.

Sanofi-Aventis agreed to pay $109 million to resolve allegations that the company gave doctors free units of Hyalgan (an injection to relieve knee pain) to encourage those doctors to buy their product. Sanofi lowered the effective price by promising these free samples to doctors, but at the same time got inflated prices from government programs by submitting false price reports,

Endo Health Solutions Inc. and its subsidiary Endo Pharmaceuticals Inc. agreed to pay $192.7 million to resolve criminal and civil liability arising from Endo's marketing of the prescription-drug Lidoderm. As part of the agreement, Endo admitted that it intended that Lidoderm be used for unapproved indications, and that it promoted Lidoderm to healthcare providers this way.

An anesthesiologist, Scott Reuben revolutionized the way physicians provide pain relief to patients undergoing orthopedic surgery for everything from torn ligaments to degenerative hips. Now, the profession is in shambles after an investigation revealed that at least 21 of Reuben's papers were false, and that the pain drugs he touted in them may have slowed postoperative healing. Reuben's studies led to the sale of billions of dollars' worth of the potentially dangerous drugs known as COX2 inhibitors, Pfizer's Celebrex (celecoxib) and Merck's Vioxx (rofecoxib), for applications whose therapeutic benefits are now in question. Reuben was a member of Pfizer's speaker's bureau and received five independent research grants from the company.

Reuben, in his now-discredited research, attempted to convince orthopedic surgeons to shift from the first generation of nonsteroidal anti-inflammatory drugs (NSAIDs) to the newer, proprietary COX2 inhibitors, such as Vioxx, Celebrex, and Pfizer's Bextra (valdecoxib). He claimed that using such drugs in combination with the Pfizer anticonvulsant Neurontin (gabapentin), and later Lyrica (pregabalin), prior to and during surgery could be effective in decreasing postoperative pain and reduce the use of addictive painkillers, such as morphine, during recovery.

Americans now spend a staggering $200 billion a year on prescription drugs, and that figure is growing at a rate of about 12 percent a year. Drugs are the fastest-growing part of the national health-care bill which itself is rising at an alarming rate. The increase in drug spending reflects, in almost equal parts, the facts that people are taking a lot more drugs than they used to, that those drugs are more likely to be expensive new ones instead of older, cheaper ones, and that the prices of the most heavily prescribed drugs are routinely increased, at episodes several times a year.

Pharmaceutical companies are primarily marketing machines used to sell drugs of sometimes uncertain benefit in many instances. This industry uses its wealth and power to label every institution that might stand in its way, including the US Congress, the FDA, academic medical centers, and the medical profession itself. Most of its marketing efforts are focused on influencing doctors, since they must write the prescriptions.

A physician got an inside look at this shadowy mess while examining drug company internal documents as an expert witness in a case against a pharmaceutical company. The voluminous amounts of documents he was given access to show serious misrepresentation of both the effectiveness and safety of certain drugs, with published articles making the research appear positive, while negative secondary outcomes were deleted. In 2005, Dr. John Ioannidis, an epidemiologist at Ioannina School of Medicine, in Greece, showed that there is less than a 50 percent chance that the results of any randomly chosen scientific paper will be true.

One common scheme by pharmaceutical manufacturers has been to market or promote their drugs to physicians for an off-label or unapproved use. Although physicians may prescribe a drug for an off-label use, pharmaceutical companies violate federal law, including the False Claims Act, when they market, promote or encourage physicians to use their drugs in an off-label or non-FDA approved manner. Pharmaceutical companies that have engaged in illegal off-label marketing or promotion of their drugs have paid the Government hundreds of millions of dollars as a result of Federal False Claims Act cases. Pharmaceutical companies have also been known to provide financial inducements to insurance companies and Group Purchasing Organizations to place their drugs on that insurer's preferred drug formulary, which can substantially increase the sales volume for those drugs.

Whistleblower cases brought under Federal and State False Claims Acts have been particularly effective in combating false and fraudulent claims by pharmaceutical manufacturers. According to publicly available data, well over $19 billion has been collected from pharmaceutical companies for various pricing, billing and marketing schemes that violate the Federal and State False Claims Acts. President Trump has recently stated that "big pharma" is now going to have to address the high drug prices, and he is demanding change. Hopefully, patients and physicians will back him in this endeavor.

Health care consumers need to identify these health care fraudsters and report them to attempt to salvage the health care system. People need to remember that he/she could receive a monetary reward for being a whistle blower.

Whistle blowers are people who expose unethical or illegal wrongdoing within companies by reporting it internally to superiors or externally to the media, government authorities, or specialized attorneys. They can be either current or past employees (insiders), or outside individuals who are familiar with the unlawful conduct, and are not required to be U.S. citizens. If you properly report Medicare fraud, you may be entitled to a significant whistleblower reward.

8. Medical Transport Fraud

Individuals should be aware of ambulance fraud. Many individuals do not realize that ambulance fraud can make a significant sum of money for an ambulance company. An ambulance is a vehicle for transportation of ill or injured people to, from or between places of treatment for an illness or injury, and in some instances will also provide out of hospital medical care to the patient. The word is often associated with road going emergency ambulances, which form part of an emergency medical service, administering emergency care to those with acute medical problems.

The term ambulance does, however, extend to a wider range of vehicles other than those with flashing warning lights and sirens. The term also includes a large number of non-urgent ambulances, which are for transport of patients without an immediate acute condition (see below: Functional types) and a wide range of urgent and non-urgent vehicles, including trucks, vans, bicycles, motorbikes, station wagons, buses, helicopters, fixed-wing aircraft, boats, and even hospital ships.

The U.S. Department of Health and Human Services has identified ambulance service as one of the biggest areas of overuse and abuse in Medicare as exemplified by ambulance companies billing millions of dollars for trips by patients who can walk, sit, stand or even drive their own cars.

Medical transport services are sometimes necessary, but be aware that some ambulance companies are inappropriately billing Medicare billions of dollars each year. These suspect medical transport companies may bill for services that you may not have received; such as oxygen, cardiac monitoring, etc.

An investigation by the Inspector General's office detected Medicare payments for potentially fraudulent ambulance rides of $54 million in the first half of 2012. During the year, Medicare Part B paid $5.8 billion for ambulance transportation, double what it paid ten years earlier. The investigators found approximately $24 million in payments by Medicare were not for rides valid under the program requirements.

Additionally, Medicare paid $30 million for transportation where there is no evidence that services were provided to the patient at either the pick-up or drop-off location. If the amounts are extrapolated out to a full year, that would be more than $100 million lost to Medicare fraud in this area alone. The problem was not limited to one company or geography.

Medicare ambulance claims, just like everything involved with Medicare, must meet certain requirements to be considered valid ambulance transport claims. The main factor is the transport must be considered "medically necessary" under Federal Law. To do this, two specific criteria must be met: The use of other transportation methods is contraindicated by the condition of the individual requiring care. The individual's medical condition must require the level and type of service reported to have been provided and billed.

Medicare pays for different levels of ambulance services, including air transport (fixed-wing and rotary-wing transport). These levels of service are differentiated by the qualifications and training of the crew and the equipment and supplies available on a vehicle that allows for treatment of more complex medical conditions. The rotary wing air ambulance may be necessary because the beneficiary's condition requires rapid transport to a treatment facility, and either great distances or other obstacles (for example, heavy traffic), preclude such rapid delivery to the nearest appropriate facility by ground ambulance.

Medicare regulations set forth medical necessity and other conditions of payment for any ambulance services. The fundamental medical necessity requirement for ambulance services, including rotary wing (helicopter) ambulance services, is that they are covered "only if they are furnished to a beneficiary whose medical condition is such that other means of transportation are contraindicated."

Air ambulance services, as opposed to ambulance services in general, are limited to instances where a patient needs immediate acute-care services in a hospital that is too far away for safe transportation by land. The illustrative list of medical services in the MCM makes it clear that air ambulance services are justified only when the patient needs emergency services that are available solely at a distant destination. The list includes the following: Intracranial bleeding requiring neurosurgical intervention; Cardiogenic shock; Burns requiring treatment in a Burn Center; Conditions requiring treatment in a Hyperbaric Oxygen Unit; Multiple severe injuries; or Life-threatening trauma.

Health Care Fraud: A Prescription for Disaster

According to evidence presented at a previous trial, the owner and operator of a Texas-based entity that purportedly provided non-emergency ambulance services to Medicare beneficiaries in the Houston area. The evidence showed that from January 2010 through December 2011, others conspired to unlawfully enrich themselves by submitting false and fraudulent claims to Medicare for ambulance services that were medically unnecessary and/or not provided. According to the further evidence presented at trial and the indictment, from approximately 1996 through September 2008, the accused individuals conspired and engaged in a scheme to defraud Medicare and Medicaid by submitting claims for payment for the transportation of patients who were not qualified to receive ambulance transportation.

Part of the problem is that it's easy to open up an ambulance company and start billing inappropriately. When a serious investigation starts the firm just shuts down, and then shows up again in some other guise, often under the name of one of the relatives of the owner. Medical providers play a role in this, too, by looking the other way when patients are being transported inappropriately, by receiving bribes from ambulance operators to refer business, or when they are faced with implicit or explicit threats from ambulance operators with organized-crime connections.

An example is that four Medicare beneficiaries received payments of up to $500 a month for riding in ambulances operated in Philadelphia. The usual model of ambulance fraud in Philadelphia involves transporting dialysis patients, who actually can travel safely by less-expensive means. One of the beneficiaries charged allegedly signed a form saying the ambulance company had transported him to a dialysis center even though he had driven himself in his Cadillac CTS.

Medicare paid $30 million for ambulance rides for which no record exists that patients got medical care at their destination, the place where they were picked up or critical information. The mystery ambulance rides are part of a bigger problem with Medicare payments for transporting patients, according to a federal audit being released Tuesday. The Department of Health and Human Services' inspector general's office also found that some urban ambulance services got paid for an average distance of more than 100 miles per ride. That contrasts with a national average of just 10 miles for urban ambulance rides.

The audit scrutinized 7.3 million ambulance rides in the first half of 2012. In addition to the mystery transports, investigators found that Medicare paid $24 million for ambulance rides that didn't meet program requirements for payment. A Russian immigrant operated his ambulance as if it was taxi service. Because Medicare reimbursed the company $400 for every round-trip to a kidney dialysis center, and each patient required three visits a week, a single customer could generate nearly $5,000 a month. The reimbursements are intended to provide service to patients who cannot walk or otherwise travel safely for treatment. Not only did patients get free rides; they received kickbacks in return for their continued patronage, prosecutors said.

Common instances of ambulance fraud may include: Billing for medically unnecessary ambulance transport: Submitting a claim for a transport that was not life-threatening or otherwise routine (e.g. scheduled radiation treatment for cancer patients). Ambulance transport "up coding occurs by falsely changing the severity of the medical necessity of a transport from "non-emergency" to "emergency" to receive a higher payment. Also billing for services not rendered during transport occurs frequently. Fabricating services and/or supplies to increase billing also occurs.

Participating in unlawful agreements/scams with health care facilities: e.g. providing ambulance transport at a lower cost in order to receive more "emergency" referrals is another fraudulent action. Transporting more than one patient at once occurs to increase revenues. Having patients ride in the front seat of the ambulance is not uncommon. Have patients ride in stretchers even though they were able to walk as well as taking patients to pick up food while billing as a dialysis clinic visit.

One scheme involved more than $3.6 million in fraudulent claims submitted to Medicare. The defendants conspired to defraud Medicare by recruiting patients who could walk and could travel safely by means other than ambulance and who therefore were not eligible for ambulance transportation under Medicare requirements. The defendants, and others acting on their behalf, falsified reports to make it appear that the patients needed to be transported by ambulance when the defendants knew that the patients could be transported safely by other means and that many of them walked to the ambulance for transport.

The defendants, themselves, or through others, paid illegal kickbacks to the patients as part of a scheme. The defendants billed Medicare for these ambulance services as if those services were medically necessary and, as a result of the fraudulent billing, the Medicare program sustained losses of more than $1.5 million for this medically unnecessary method of transportation.

Throughout the first half of 2015, a number of fraud cases and investigations have focused on ambulance services, particularly for non-emergency transportation. In some instances, these cases have implications for both ambulance companies as well as hospitals. Meanwhile, in Florida, one ambulance company and nine hospitals collectively paid $7.5 million to settle false claims allegations that the providers conspired to provide unnecessary emergency transportation to healthy patients.

Authorities allege that between 2007 and 2011, a company, billed for emergency ambulance services, which were not actually emergencies. Medicare pays substantially higher pay outs for emergency ambulance reimbursement than for non-emergency calls. The resolution of some of these lawsuits means that millions of taxpayer dollars that were used to reimburse false claims by the ambulance service have been recovered.

Health care consumers need to identify these health care fraudsters and report them to attempt to salvage the health care system. People need to remember that he/she could receive a monetary reward for being a whistle blower.

Whistle blowers are people who expose unethical or illegal wrongdoing within companies by reporting it internally to superiors or externally to the media, government authorities, or specialized attorneys. They can be either current or past employees (insiders), or outside individuals who are familiar with the unlawful conduct, and are not required to be U.S. citizens. If you properly report Medicare fraud, you may be entitled to a significant whistleblower reward.

9. Workman's Compensation Fraud

Workman's compensation was originally designed to provide assistance to an injured worker. An injured worker's medical expenses were paid for and the injured worker would receive some pay to offset the loss of income. Thid philosophy has changed with some workman's compensation companies.

A patient should be aware that fraud addressed to an injured worker can occur on occasion. In some instances, it is the insurance company which commits the fraud. If a patient suspects deception he/she should consult an attorney. Workers' compensation generally is supposed to provide injured workers with full medical insurance coverage, rehabilitation costs, and two-thirds of regular weekly pay during disability caused by a workplace injury (or a specified death benefit in case of fatality) without regard to the fault of workers or employers.

If a patient is injured on the job and makes a workers' comp claim, the patient must be medically evaluated and treated by doctors who are approved by a patient employer's insurance company. In worker's compensation cases, there is always the possibility that a doctor will find nothing wrong with a worker's comp client. Treating doctors are very important witnesses in every kind of injury case.

Workers Compensation Insurance is a state-run program. A patient's employer, and most of the time a patient, pay premiums each month (patients comes out in payroll taxes), and those premiums are set according to the degree of hazard and the number and costs of claims a patient's employer experiences on average in a patient's state. They desire to keep these premiums, and their costs, low and this can lead to conflicts over coverage, allowance and sometimes even the handling of a patient's claim.

State workers' compensation laws are administered by what is usually called the "workers' comp commission" in each state, appointed by the governor. The commission decides disputed cases when employers contest workers' claims that their injuries are work-related and deserving of compensation. Administrative law judges hear evidence in disputed cases, and their decisions can be appealed to the state commission for review.

Navigating the workers' compensation medical process can add even more discomfort to a painful work injury. Each state has its own rules and regulations regarding workers' comp claims, but one rule is common to all: Injured workers seeking benefits must be evaluated and diagnosed by workers' compensation doctors hired by the employer's insurance company.

Treating doctors, and what their opinions are of utmost importance to a workers compensation client. That's because only a doctor can testify about the nature and extent of injury as well as causation. In workers comp cases, causation refers to a doctor's opinion as to whether the injury is work-related. Doctors have various reasons for deciding to work for an insurance company, and his/her or her ultimate goal is money.

Virtually all state regulations permit a patient to be treated by a patient own doctor, but a patient's claim is highly dependent on the medical opinion of the doctor(s) a patient chooses from the insurance company's approved list. Doctors have various reasons for deciding to work for an insurance company, but like most people in the workforce, their goal is a paycheck. Whether they are seeking to augment their private practices or are retired and need additional income, most are financially motivated. Workers' compensation doctors know insurance companies don't like spending money on diagnostics. They are expensive and complicate the entire claim.

As a result, many insurance company approved doctors are more likely to treat injuries with pain medication. Medications are less expensive than an MRI. Too often doctors don't believe patients' accounts of their pain and discomfort. To remain upon the list for workers' comp referrals, some doctors may classify patients as malingerers, rather than diagnosing real pain issues. That's why second opinions are so valuable.

There is no such thing as a true independent medical examination (IME). Doctors hired to perform IMEs are usually paid by the same workers' comp insurance company handling a patient claim. In most cases, the adjuster working a patient claim chooses the doctor a patient will be required to see. If requested by the insurance company, a patient must submit to an IME. A patient refusal may allow the adjuster to deny a patient's claim. Most doctors who perform IMEs have little incentive to take the necessary time to study all the medical documentation related to a patient claim. Fees are based on the number of patients examined, not on the time spent on each case. Essentially this behavior is fraudulent.

Nurse case managers are registered nurses whose job is to facilitate communication between the doctor and the insurance company. A patient may have a nurse case manager assigned to help a patient with a patient's claim. The nurse may present herself as a patient advocate who is acting in a patient's best interest. Although most nurses are honest and hard-working, do not forget that she is employed by the insurance company.

In most states a patient can refuse to have the nurse in the examination room with a patient while a patient is seeing the doctor. A patient should seek a second opinion if a patient feel the workers' compensation doctor a patient chose isn't addressing a patient's medical issues. Most workers' comp insurance companies permit an injured worker to have a second evaluation from another doctor on their approved list.

While second opinions may seem helpful, the other doctors rendering those opinions are under the same conflict of interest as the primary one. After a specified time, usually 30 days or more after filing a patient's claim, a patient will be permitted to have an evaluation and treatment from a physician a patient choose, whether on the approved list or not.

Not seeking treatment right away tells insurance that a patient wasn't hurt that seriously. A consultation visit regarding a claim will always be paid for by the employer or a patient's self-insured employer. A patient's employer may recommend a physician who will save them money by minimizing a patient injury. An injury on the job can cause anxiety, depression, and even a post-traumatic stress disorder. If a patient is not experiencing these symptoms, the insurance company implies that here is nothing wrong with the patient. The patient is deemed "normal" after the accident. An injured worker should talk to a workers' compensation lawyer and get a second medical opinion. Too many worker's compensation doctors would rather satisfy the workman's compensation insurance adjustor rather than provide a patient with good medical care.

Employers and insurance claims adjusters commonly send injured workers for second opinion exams by an "independent" doctor. As mentioned this is called an IME as mentioned, which stands for an insurance medical exam, or independent medical exam. The independent insurance doctors are selected by a patient's employer or a workers compensation insurance company, and in some instances, they are paid to find nothing wrong with a seriously injured worker.

If a patient receives a letter requesting a patient's presence at an independent medical examination, a patient is required by law to attend. The IME gives a patient's employer or its insurance company an opportunity to have a patient examined by a doctor of their choice. If a patient does not attend this examination, the patient faces losing worker's compensation benefits. It is common for an independent medical examination to conclude that a patient's condition is not work-related or that a patient can go back to work without restrictions. Many IME consultations find no evidence of injury. Insurance companies use the same doctors repeatedly, because they know what to expect from these individuals. Some of these doctors make a career out of testifying for insurance companies.

If a patient has been injured on the job, the insurance company may hire a private investigator to watch a patient. The goal of this action is to do try to observe a patient doing something a patient's doctor told a patient not to do or something a patient told a patient's doctor that the patient could not do. A video of a patient doing something a patient told a patient's doctor he/she could not do is unfavorable to a patient's case. Surveillance is most commonly ordered when a hearing or settlement mediation is approaching.

Private investigators need an opportunity to "pick a patient up." That's what they call it when they start following a patient. Commonly they will do this at a patient house or at a patient's doctor's visit. Because the insurance company knows when a patient will have a doctor's appointment it is easy for them to tell the private investigator where and when they will be able to find the patient in question. Frequently, investigators will park down the street and watch a patient's house. A patient should not be in the yard doing yard work if a patient's doctor told a patient not to so. Taking out the trash is another investigator favorite. They want to catch a patient taking out trash when a patient has lifting restrictions and assumes it must have been over the doctor's prescribed limits.

When a doctor releases a patient to return to work, with or without restrictions, a patient's employer or its workers' compensation insurance carrier must send a patient a form entitled a Notice of Ability to Return to Work with the doctor's release before they can offer a patient a return to work. If a patient receives a return to work offer before a patient receives a Notice of Ability to Return to Work form, the patient must contact a workers' compensation lawyer immediately.

The meat and poultry industry have been alleged on occasion to administer workers' compensation programs by steadily failing to recognize and report claims, delaying claims, denying claims, and threatening and taking reprisals against workers who file claims for compensation for workplace injuries. An administrative law judge previously sued the Arkansas Workers' Compensation Commission for wrongful dismissal after the commission fired her. The judge said her firing was a response to pressure from businesses because of her decisions favoring injured workers.

Insurance companies frequently contest workers' compensation claimed for injuries which are musculoskeletal as separate from injuries, which are traumatic and visible. If it's not something obvious with witnesses, the insurance company may state that it is not a job-related injury and denies the workers' compensation claim. These companies have an incentive to deny claims or to direct workers toward their regular medical insurance program.

Many workers are fearful of losing their jobs if they request compensation for a workplace injury. Such retaliation is unlawful in every state (except Alabama, which allows employers to fire workers for filing compensation claims). Most states permit employers to have a worker claiming compensation see a company selected physician in addition to the employee's own physician, with provisions for a third opinion in case of a dispute between physicians. Workman's compensation doctors do not need special training to evaluated injured workers and only need to have a state license and be authorized in a specialty.

Most injured workers do not realize that with respect to workers' compensation, it is not enough to prove that a worker was hurt on the job. A patient has to show that he/she suffered an accidental injury at the time he/she was hurt or that an injury was caused by a specific traumatic event or that a patient suffered from an occupational disease.

Federal workers' compensation is entirely different from state's workers' compensation, and there are few attorneys who have specialized experience in the field. The U.S. government provides benefits to civilian federal workers who become injured or ill because of their job duties. The Federal Employees Compensation Act (FECA) is the governing law over federal workers' compensation, is administered by the U.S. Department of Labor, Office of Workers' Compensation Programs (OWCP).

If a patient is injured at work, a patient will initially file a claim with the OWCP, and a claims examiner will be assigned to review the patient's file. In cases of traumatic injuries, a patient may receive a continuation of full pay for the first 45 days of disability. Otherwise, if a patient sustains a disabling, job-related injury or illness, a patient may be eligible to receive two-thirds of the patient's pre-disability wages, or three fourths if an injured worker has dependents.

If a patient suffers from a specific job-related permanent partial impairment, such as the loss of the use of a limb, after a patient has exhausted temporary total disability benefits, a patient may be entitled to schedule award. A schedule award consists of monetary payments for a prescribed number of weeks set by statutes and regulations. There are also cases where a patient may have a pre-existing injury or medical condition, which is aggravated by an event that occurred on the job. A key difference between federal and state workers' compensation is the matter of apportionment. In states' workers' compensation, an aggravated injury or condition may only be partially covered by a patient's employing agency.

In contrast, federal workers' compensation claims only take into account the employee's current state of well-being. If a patient had suffered from a back injury years ago, but heavy lifting required by a patient's current job duty aggravates the condition, then the OWCP may cover all of patient required medical needs, rather than just a portion of it.

MMI (Maximum Medical Improvement) is addressed to any worker injured who is actively being treated and symptomatic for a duration of more than six months and is required to be rated for permanent impairment utilizing the AMA Guides To Impairment. Different states will use different editions of these guidelines. In Colorado, this book provides workers' compensation physicians charts that assign a numeric impairment rating utilizing both diagnosis and range of motion determinations.

These ratings then convert to money benefits required to be paid to the worker under the law. A rating on simply a strained back, with some limited range of motion can mean upward of $60,000 or more in money paid to a worker (depending on age and pay rate). However, the Guide often requires both active care and ongoing symptoms for a duration of greater than six months in order for a rating to be given.

Doctors whose source of revenue depends on keeping employers and insurance companies content are finding more and more resourceful ways to justify releasing worker's compensation patients back to work just shy of the six-month mark in an effort to cheat the employee out of a much deserved and substantial money recovery. The initial denial of a claim is a major issue in workers' compensation cases. Insurance companies are under pressure from their clients to keep premium costs as low as possible. They carefully scrutinize claims for opportunities to deny or reduce benefits. Because of this behavior, the injured worker should have the right to have a video recording of compelled medical exams as a matter of an injured worker's right.

This action might reduce insurance company fraud.

10. Pill Mill Fraud

A pain management clinic (in the general legal definition) is a facility providing pain treatment options or that has at least one doctor licensed to prescribe controlled medication for pain. Pain clinics are subject to legal rules and standards, such as being licensed, being subject to inspection by the board and the state, employing licensed staff, etc. Prescription pain medication is regulated by federal law, so doctors who prescribe it without a legitimate medical purpose or outside the usual course of medical practice can be charged with drug trafficking. Pill mills are essentially places where doctors hand out prescription drugs.

A Pill Mill is essentially a term used primarily by local and state investigators to describe a doctor, clinic or pharmacy that is prescribing or dispensing powerful narcotics inappropriately or for non-medical reasons. These pill mills usually: Accept cash only, do no physical exams, No medical records or x-rays are needed to be admitted to the clinic. A patient picks his/her medication. No questions about a patient's medical condition are asked. Patients may be directed to a certain pharmacy, Patients are only treated with pills. A patient gets a set number of pills, and the facility will tell a patient a specific date to return. These clinics may have security guards and there may be huge masses of people waiting to see the doctor. By contrast, in many "pain clinics," walk-ins are the only method of intake. The office is understaffed. No referral is required and little or no examination or work-up is done.

A legitimate practice will only accept patients who have health insurance, whereas most "pill mills" will see patients for cash payments without any health insurance. This difference is a giveaway, since most insurance companies will actually require that physicians who provide care to their patients meet certain standards and be board-certified in the specialty. Otherwise, care and visits will not be authorized. To be more specific, a "pill mill" according to the State of Florida is a doctor's office, clinic, or health care facility that routinely conspires in the prescribing and dispensing of controlled substances outside the scope of the prevailing standards of medical practice within the community or violates the laws of the state of Florida regarding the prescribing or dispensing of controlled prescription drugs.

Signs that a facility may actually be a pill mill as previously mentioned include not requiring a physical exam, X-rays or medical records before being prescribed drugs, being able to pick your preferred medication, being directed to "their" specific pharmacy, and treating pain solely with pills. Pill mills also tend to open and close very suddenly, as an attempt to evade law enforcement.

The term "pill mill" is the nickname given for the illegitimate pain clinics that have sprung up in strip malls and office parks nationwide over the past few years. These alleged pain management centers tend to occupy unmarked office spaces or storefronts, may display a misleading or false business name and have armed security guards patrolling the clinic's lobby. Armed security guards are needed to prevent thieves from robbing the pill mill cache of drugs. The clinics are employed by unlicensed doctors who prescribe massive amounts of powerful narcotic medications to anyone who walks into the clinic off the street. Although they exist nationwide, most pill mills are located in Texas, Kentucky and Florida due to the states' previous looser restrictions on prescription-drug monitoring.

All pill mills operate in the same fashion: no medical records, x-rays, or examinations are needed; pain is treated only with prescription medication; patients can request whatever medication they want with no questions asked; only cash is accepted; prescriptions can only be retrieved from their pharmacy, and patients must return on a specific date to obtain more prescriptions. The idea is to get patients hooked on these drugs to ensure the sale of more drugs and help physicians quickly profit. The clinics tend to shut down and open up in new locations to avoid getting caught by law enforcement and face legal prosecution and pill mill owners are hard to trace since clinics are registered with absent doctors or stolen identities. The closing down of many "pill mills" has resulted in "patients" willing to drive a long way to continue receiving prescriptions from other doctors.

Today, pain specialists rarely prescribe strong opioids for chronic pain unless it's cancer-related. From late 1980s through early 2000s, physicians tried to improve the way they treated chronic pain by prescribing opioids for more people. They believed that by taking the highly addictive drugs only as prescribed for pain control, patients wouldn't become addicted. There are growing rates of addiction to heroin. The reason is that the less-expensive opioid is commonly turned to by addicts for cost reasons or when their pill mill gets shut down.

An opioid is any "opium-like" substance that binds to the opioid receptors in the human brain, which includes heroin but also substances like hydrocodone, oxycodone and morphine found in prescription painkillers. These drugs at certain doses can stop a patient's ability to breathe, which may ultimately result in death of a patient. Drug mills cause drug addiction and destruction to livelihoods, families, and communities. Such characteristics can be far easier to spot and investigate when prescription-drug databases are used as a mandate. Other states have had vast success in reducing illegal prescriptions when implementing the mandatory use of their state prescription drug database. Medical board support for the mandatory use of prescription-drug database will go a long way to help take drugs off the streets, protect patients and identify impaired or drug-dealing doctors."

Certain legislation, like Tennessee's Intractable Pain Treatment Act, on the other hand has been accused of establishing a realm where pill mills can flourish. Put into effect in 2001, the Tennessee measure was meant to make drugs, like the newly developed oxycodone, more accessible to patients with cancer and intractable pain. What the act ended up facilitating was an "explosion in use" of prescription painkillers in locales like Sullivan County (which saw 11 pain clinics emerge to meet the demand.

It is against Federal law for a doctor to prescribe pain medication without a legitimate medical purpose or "outside the usual course of medical practice." For example, if a prescription is deemed as not valid, a doctor could be charged with drug trafficking. This is a felony with the possibility of up to life in prison. It is also illegal to practice or prescribe a medicine without a license.

Pill mills can have a negative impact on some communities. As mentioned previously, a pill mill is an operation in which a doctor, clinic or pharmacy prescribes and/or dispenses narcotics without a legitimate medical purpose. In a typical Kentucky town, complaints started coming in from business owners neighboring a pill mill, complaining that the parking lots overflow with drug seekers, tailgating while waiting for their appointments and snorting pills outside the buildings.

These are just a few typical signs of the establishment of a pill mill in a community, Remember that a pill mill is an operation in which a doctor, clinic or pharmacy prescribes and/or dispenses narcotics without a legitimate medical purpose. Unlike a typical clinic, it is strictly a cash business. There is no insurance plan and no individualized treatment. If a patient's pain could be eased with physical therapy, injection therapy, braces or surgery, it would not be a treatment option offered in a pill mill.

Recently, the DEA conducted Operation "Pilluted', the largest pharmaceutical drug investigation of all time, where across four southern states over 140 people, mostly doctors and pharmacists, were arrested for their participation in dispensing narcotics without a legitimate medical purpose. Local and state authorities across the Deep South have been working closely with the Drug Enforcement Administration and other federal agencies over the past 15 months to stem the flow of prescription medications flooding the streets. Officials with the DEA New Orleans Field Division said the extensive investigation, dubbed Operation Pilluted, led to the arrest of 22 doctors and pharmacists and 280 other individuals across Arkansas, Alabama, Louisiana and Mississippi.

Agents executed 21 search warrants across the four states during the course of the investigation. Those warrants led to the seizure of 51 vehicles, 202 weapons and $404,828 in cash. Agents also executed 73 seizure warrants that netted more than $11 million in currency and $6.7 million in real property. However, as clinics dispensing oxycodone and hydrocodone are being dismantled, new ones continue to spring up.

Buprenorphine, branded under Suboxone or Subutex, is the latest narcotic being churned out by networks of shady clinics. It also happens to be the very drug that is supposed to help opiate users kick their habit. Suboxone Film contains buprenorphine, an opioid that can cause physical dependence with chronic use. Physical dependence is not the same as addiction.

Kentucky state officials also found the use of buprenorphine increased 241% since 2012, which is the same year many of the pill mills selling oxycodone met their demise. That same report found one user who was doctor shopping, obtaining prescriptions from nine different prescribers. Buprenorphine came on to the scene where a cash for pills market was already set, and where practices like doctor shopping through networks of certain doctors were in full swing.

Some doctors now prescribe buprenorphine and other opioids in combination with benzodiazepines. The combination of opioids and benzodiazepines greatly increases the risk of a fatal overdose. When the DEA cracked down on pill mills and other systems of prescription-drug abuse, it inadvertently caused users to flock to a ready and waiting supply of cheap heroin. Hence the four-fold increase in heroin-related mortality from 2000-2013, reported by the CDC. It's worth noting, that most of this mortality spike occurred after 2010, around the time prescription painkillers became more tightly con-trolled. Many opiate users seek Suboxone to ward off withdrawal symptoms in the event their source runs dry; they run out of money, or are sincerely trying to kick.

In Kentucky, prior to the initial prescribing or dispensing of certain classes of controlled substance, the practitioner shall: Obtain a complete medical history and conduct a physical examination of the patient and document the information in the patient's medical record; Query a physician prescribing database (called KASPER) for all available data about the patient; Make a written treatment plan stating the objectives of the treatment and further diagnostic examinations required; Discuss the risks and benefits from the use of controlled substances with the patient, including the risk of tolerance and drug dependence; and Obtain written consent for the treatment.

In addition, a practitioner must periodically monitor the course of treatment and query the state physician prescribing database no less than once every three months before issuing any new prescription refills for the controlled substances. The practitioner must also create and maintain detailed records regarding the patient, and the controlled substances pre-scribed. The bill also mandates that each health-care professional licensing board in the Commonwealth establish regulations regarding controlled substances, including establishing mandatory prescribing and dispensing standards, prohibiting a practitioner from dispensing greater than a forty-eight-hour supply of certain controlled substances, and establishing procedures for suspending a practitioner's license to protect patients and the public.

The nationwide surge in deaths now places prescription drug over-doses as the second-leading cause of accidental death behind traffic crashes and painkillers as the top narcotic contributing to death. A recent National Drug Assessment study shows that prescription narcotics are the second most abused drug (behind marijuana).

Lawmakers and law enforcers have been cracking down recently on clinics, as well as doctors and pharmacies that illegally or irresponsibly dispense prescription narcotics. These clinics sell prescription drugs to those who have no medical need of them, or in excessive amounts, and have directly contributed to many of the recent restrictions that have been placed upon the distribution and availability of prescription drugs. Although they can be found all over the country, they have made most notable headlines in Florida, Kentucky and Texas,

Federal law empowers state medical board inspectors to enter any clinic and inspect its books and procedures. It is important for people to be vigilant when buying prescription drugs from clinics and pharmacies. Some of the most common prescription drugs sold in drug mills include Vicodin, Percocet, and OxyContin. States that have conducted crackdowns on drug mills have experienced considerably fewer deaths from drug overdoses. Crackdowns on drug mills are some of the most effective ways for states to reduce prescription and narcotic drug overdose death rates. Pill mill clinics accept cash only. Cash leaves no paper trail for the reporting of income. The patient might not even be seen by a physician or have no physical exam during the visit. In a pill mill, no diagnostic X-rays are ordered. There are no referrals for physical therapy, but only a monthly supply of a deadly combo of drugs.

The Hippocratic Oath clearly states, "I will neither give a deadly drug to anybody who asked for it, nor will I make a suggestion to this effect." A study conducted by the Centers for Disease Control, and Prevention stated that a relatively small number of doctors were responsible for a large proportion of painkiller prescriptions. Dealers obtain the maximum prescription 240 pills and then turn around and sell the pills. On average, a 30-milligram Oxycodone pill has a street value of about $10 to $12.00. Otherwise, the pill runs $1.42 at a pharmacy, according to a Johns Hopkins University website.

A county in Florida established the following pain clinic rule with respect to opioid prescribing: Requirements of the new law include: Pain clinics must be owned by a doctor, group of doctors or registered under the Agency for Health Care Administration. The Department of Health will conduct annual inspections and document any violations. A physical exam must be performed the same day the prescription is prescribed.

If a doctor prescribes more than a 72-hour supply of medicine for pain, the reason must be documented in the patient's medical record. A doctor cannot dispense more than a 72-hour supply for patients who pay with cash, check or credit card instead of insurance. Doctors must use counterfeit resistant prescription blanks. While many pain clinics and doctors take their position very seriously and only prescribe drugs after carefully determining their patients' needs, many others are simply getting rich off of other people's drug addiction.

The number of people dying because of prescription and narcotic drugs overdose has risen significantly and drug mills are a major source of this problem. Below are the states that had the most providers prescribing 3,000 prescriptions for Schedule 2 controlled substances in 2012 in Medicare Part D, per ProPublica: Florida: 52 providers, Tennessee: 25 providers, North Carolina: 15 providers, Ohio:15 providers, Georgia:14 providers, Pennsylvania: 12 providers, Alabama:12 providers, Kentucky: 11 providers, Oklahoma,:, Arizona, Arkansas and Texas 9

There are different ways to curb prescription drug abuse. The first way has already been taking place across the country, which is to arrest and charge doctors that operate pill mills. It is also necessary to more closely monitor patients who use prescription painkillers, through better regulations at clinics or doctors' offices, or through a prescription-drug database. Only a small number of pain clinics actually fill a very large amount of oxycodone prescriptions compared to those filled at pharmacies.

While legitimate pain management clinics do exist to serve those with chronic pain or terminal illness, other unscrupulous clinics, called pill mills, merely serve only as drug traffickers. Remember that the common characteristics of pill mills as previously mentioned include: cash only, no insurance; no appointments; armed guards; little or no medical records; grossly inadequate physical examinations; and large prescription doses of narcotics that exceed the boundaries of acceptable medical care. The drug contract patient -doctor agreements may require patients to submit to blood or urine drug tests, fill their prescriptions at a single pharmacy or refuse to accept pain medication from any other doctor. If patients don't follow the rules, the agreements often state that doctors may drop them from their practice.

Pain is such a nebulous pathology that it's hard to point a finger and rightfully accuse a pain management doctor for harming a patient by pre-scribing the medications. It could very well be that the patient really does need that drug in order to function in life, especially in chronic pain patients. However, it could be that patient is an addict, and the doctor is reinforcing that behavior for the business. For the latter case, it is a criminal act. However, it's very difficult to prove such intentions.

Before a pain clinic accepts a chronic pain patient, a patient should have to fulfill basic criteria: Be over 21 years old, have pain greater than 3 months in duration and be anticipated to continue on pain management indefinitely. A patient must have a verifiable (laboratory tests, CT or MRI evaluations) and pathological problem that is severe enough to qualify he/she as a chronic pain patient. Furthermore, a patient must agree to pursue therapies that can alleviate their pain (e.g. physical therapy, behavioral therapy, weight loss, regular exercise and smoking cessation).

Patient intake documentation must be completed and verified. The patient must furthermore agree to regular drug testing. Pain medicine is absolutely not about prescribing opioids. It's about treating the whole patient. Anyone who suspects a pail mill should report it to local authorities. Pain management is a delicate balance. It's difficult to help a patient regain his or her quality of life and keep them from becoming addicted. However, this action could save a life. If you suspect pill mill activity contact your DEA office.

Health care consumers need to identify these health care fraudsters and report them to attempt to salvage the health care system. People need to remember that he/she could receive a monetary reward for being a whistle blower.

Whistle blowers are people who expose unethical or illegal wrongdoing within companies by reporting it internally to superiors or externally to the media, government authorities, or specialized attorneys. They can be either current or past employees (insiders), or outside individuals who are familiar with the unlawful conduct, and are not required to be U.S. citizens. If you properly report Medicare fraud, you may be entitled to a significant whistleblower reward.

11. Addiction Medicine Fraud

Chronic opioid therapy (defined as greater than three months on opioids) is a common practice for those with non-cancer pain, cancer survivors with treatment-related pain, and individuals with cancer undergoing disease-modifying therapy with a survival that can be for a year or more. Drugs are chemicals that have a profound impact on the neurochemical balance in the brain. The risk of addiction, depression, central hypogonadism, sleep-disordered breathing, impaired wound healing, infections, cognitive impairment, falls, non-vertebral fractures, and mortality are increased in populations on long-term opioids.

Chronic pain, whether arising from bone, or any other tissue or structure, is, more often than commonly thought, the result of a mixture of pain mechanisms, and therefore, there is no simple formula available to manage chronic complex pain states. One possible explanation for the severe pain described in some patients is opioid induced hyperalgesia induced by high doses of opioids. Patients receiving chronic opioid treatment that develop paradoxical pain sensations, as well as worsening existing pain, can be diagnosed as suffering from opioid-induced hyperalgesia. As the worldwide population expands so too does the proportion of patients who experience pain that requires a strong opioid.

Opioid-induced hyperalgesia (OIH) is a phenomenon associated with the long-term use of opioids such as morphine, hydrocodone, oxycodone, and methadone. This entity may mimic addiction. Identifying the development of hyperalgesia is of great clinical importance since patients receiving opioids to relieve pain may paradoxically experience more pain as a result of treatment. As a result, he/she takes more pain medication and subsequently appears to be addicted. Ketamine has been shown to be significantly beneficial in patients who require large amounts of opioid medications or exhibit some degree of opioid tolerance. Methadone is also effective in reducing high-dose opioid OIH.

The clinical use of opioids is further complicated by an increasingly deleterious profile of side effects beyond addiction, including tolerance and opioid-induced hyperalgesia (OIH), where OIH is defined as an increased sensitivity to already painful stimuli. This paradoxical state of increased nociception results from acute and long-term exposure to opioids, and appears to develop in a substantial subset of patients using opioids. As more opioids are prescribed, especially to treat chronic nonmalignant pain, OIH becomes more of a relevant and significant issue.

In the last decade, a significant number of preclinical studies have investigated the factors that modulate OIH development as well as the cellular and molecular mechanisms underlying OIH. Several factors have been shown to influence OIH including the genetic background and sex differences of experimental animals as well as the opioid regimen. Mu opioid receptor variants and interactions with different proteins were shown to be important. Furthermore, at the cellular level, both neurons and glia play a major role in OIH development.

People who are suffering emotionally use drugs to escape from their problems, and this can lead to drug abuse and addiction. While progress is being made in treating patients with CRPS (Complex Regional Pain Syndrome), it is important to remember that the goals of care are always to: 1) perform a comprehensive diagnostic evaluation, 2) be prompt and aggressive in treatment interventions, 3) assess and reassess the patient's clinical and psychological status, 4) be consistently supportive, and 5) strive for the maximal amount of pain relief and function-al improvement.

The annual number of US deaths from a prescription-opioid overdose quadrupled between 1999 and 2010 and in 2010 alone reached 16,651. Deaths from an opioid overdose have now surpassed the historic death toll from another drug-related epidemic - anesthesia mortality. Repeated, or chronic, use of opioids induces adaptive or allosteric changes that modify neuronal circuitry and create an altered normality. Patients receiving long-term opioid therapy often transitioned to chronic use after starting opioids.

Ongoing opioid analgesic use in patients suffering from chronic non-malignant pain (CNMP) has been associated with the development of opioid misuse, abuse, addiction, and overdose. Some physicians are afraid to prescribe scheduled drugs because of the possibility of causing addiction. Chronic pain, whether arising from viscera, bone, or any other tissue or structure, is, more often than commonly thought, the result of a mixture of pain mechanisms, and therefore there is no simple formula available to manage chronic complex pain states. It has been shown previously that the risk of true addiction in chronic pain patients was approximately 0.3%. Accurate anatomical diagnosis can be provided in only 15% of the patients utilizing traditional medical technology. The question of, "Why not relief?" should be raised in our society on a daily basis.

It is imperative to understand the true nature of pain by separating the myth of psychological pain from the reality of organic pain and manage it appropriately utilizing all available means, not only narcotics and interventional technology, but also behavioral therapy. Prescription monitoring programs and using urine toxicology to monitor opioid use may decrease opioid abuse. CRPS patients may request opioids to control the severe pain.

Addiction is a chronic relapsing brain disease. Brain imaging shows that addiction severely alters the brain's areas critical to decision-making, learning and memory, and behavior control, which may help to explain the compulsive and destructive behaviors of addiction. An addiction is a recurring problem by an individual to engage in some specific activity, despite harmful consequences to the individual's health, mental state or social life. An addiction can occur with drugs, gambling, overeating, etc. Drugs can make one euphoric. As a result, one may request more and more drugs to maintain this euphoria.

Moreover, aversion to addiction and diversion remains a potent force that shapes prescribing profiles. Addiction is a hindrance in the long-term treatment of complex regional pain syndrome (CRPS) because addiction in itself aggravates CRPS, causes stress in the sympathetic nervous system resulting in more severe sympathetic dysfunction.

Drug abuse or substance abuse, involves the repeated and excessive use of prescription or street drugs. In one way or another, almost all drugs over stimulate the pleasure center of the brain, flooding it with the neuro-transmitter dopamine which produces euphoria. That heightened sense of pleasure is so compelling that the brain wants that feeling back, repeatedly. Addiction is frequently found in people with a wide variety of mental illnesses, including anxiety disorders, unipolar and bipolar depression, schizophrenia, and borderline and other personality disorders.

Long-term pain narcotic patients should be limited to the nonaddicting pain medications (such as Stadol or Ultram) or at least to the less addicting pain medications such as Stadol or Buprenorphine

(Buprenex). Methadone may be considered in severe pain that is refractive to these drugs. Methadone can be used in the treatment of pain in addicted patients. Methadone is also an opiate that prevents users from getting high on heroin by competing with the much more potent opiates for the body's opiate receptors. Buprenorphine is another drug that is effective for the treatment of addiction and is also an analgesic.

Addiction and drug dependence occur when drugs become so important that a patient is willing to sacrifice his/her or her work, home and even the family. Once a patient's brain and body get used to the substances a patient is taking, a patient begins to require increasingly larger and more frequent doses, in order to achieve the same effect. Narcotics such as Heroin may over-stimulate the pleasure centers within the brain producing euphoric effects that cause compulsive drug-seeking behaviors. The severities of withdrawal symptoms associated with narcotics include chills, shakes, muscle pain, nausea, vomiting, and headaches and cravings. A clinician must be able to distinguish between legitimate patients in chronic pain, and individuals engaged in non-therapeutic drug seeking behavior. Physicians have for years recognized the value of opioid analgesics in relieving chronic pain.

Unfortunately, drug seekers may also request opioid analgesics. They do this by feigning illnesses, and seek controlled substances from multiple doctors and by forge prescriptions. Drug seekers may be difficult to distinguish from true chronic pain sufferers. In general, drug seekers prefer illicit drugs such as heroin and cocaine to prescription drugs. Prescription drugs, however, have advantages over illicit drugs. Third-party insurers or welfare-entitlement programs may pay for prescribed drugs. Prescription pharmaceuticals are obtained in the safety of the physician's office. Drug abuse and addiction have a devastating impact on society. Heroin use alone is responsible for the epidemic number of new cases of HIV/AIDS and hepatitis. Drug abuse is responsible for decreased job productivity and attendance, increased healthcare costs, and an escalation of domestic violence and violent crimes.

An estimated 20 percent of people in the United States have used prescription drugs for non-medical reasons. Central nervous stimulants, depressants and opioids are prescription drugs that are frequently abused. Central nervous system depressants are used to treat anxiety, panic attacks, and sleep disorders. Examples are Nembutal (pentobarbital sodium), Valium (diazepam), and Xanax (alprazolam). Long-term use can lead to physical dependence and addiction. Central nervous system stimulants are used to treat narcolepsy and the attention-deficit/hyperactivity disorder. Examples include Ritalin (methylphenidate) and Dexedrine (dextroamphetamine). Opioids, also known as narcotic analgesics are used to treat pain. Opioids are the most commonly abused prescription drugs. Examples include morphine, codeine, OxyContin (oxycodone), Vicodin (hydrocodone) and Demerol (meperidine).

One may obtain drugs by the following means: prescription forgery, by telephone (faking to be a physician's office), multiple doctors, and indiscriminate prescribing by physicians. Pain clinicians who prescribe chronic opioids are aware that there is an illicit market for opioid analgesics. For example, OxyContin can be sold for $1.00 per milligram. One 80 mg pill can be sold in the street for $80.00. Telephone scams occur when the drug seeker claims to be a patient of one of the other physicians in the on-call group, and asks for a prescription for an analgesic to last until they can see their regular physician. Sometimes, the drug seeker uses a telephone to impersonate a practicing physician. Prescription forgery is a common activity among drug seekers.

Drug seekers can modify a legitimate prescription to increase the dosage or quantity of an opioid. The easiest method is to increase the number of tablets on the prescription. Multiple episodes of noncompliance raise an alert of drug seeking behavior as well as multiple episodes of prescription loss. The patient with chemical dependency loses control over drug taking. The patient cannot take medications as prescribed. The patient repeatedly reports lost or stolen medications. The physician will notice that the drug seeker frequently requests early renewals of prescriptions. A pain physician must however, be aware that aggressive complaining about the need for more drugs may indicate inadequate pain management as opposed to drug seeking behavior.

A patient should not be allowed to suffer. It should be understood that substance abusers can suffer from chronic pain which should be treated in a humane manner. Unapproved use of opioids to treat another symptom such as sleep deprivation should not be tolerated. However, the pain management physician must objectively identify a patient's pain complaint with the appropriate medical test before prescribing an opioid. Opioid analgesics are powerful tools in the armamentarium of the pain clinician. Criminal and chemically dependent drug seekers may attempt to obtain such drugs from the physician. A pain medicine physician must therefore, use safe prescribing strategies.

A physician has no legal obligation to prescribe opioid analgesics on demand. A reasonable precaution to be taken by the pain medicine physician with an unfamiliar patient is to establish a policy of not prescribing opioid analgesics pending a complete assessment, including corroboration of the patient's history. Some patients or patient families are afraid of addiction. However, a significant number of individuals do not understand the difference between addiction and tolerance. The American Academy of Pain Medicine, the American Pain Society, and the American Society of Addiction Medicine recognize the following definitions and recommend their use.

I. Addiction

Addiction is a primary, chronic, neurobiological disease, with genetic, psychosocial, and environmental factors influencing its development and manifestations. It is characterized by behaviors that include one or more of the following: impaired control over drug use, compulsive use, continued use despite harm, and craving.

An entity termed pseudo-addiction exists, which is not true addiction. Pseudo-addiction occurs when pain is under treated. Pseudo addiction resolves when the pain resolves. Addictive behavior, on the other hand, persists in spite of increasing the patient's pain medication.

II. Physical Dependence

Physical dependence is a state of adaptation that is manifested by a drug class specific withdrawal syndrome that can be produced by abrupt cessation, rapid dose reduction, decreasing blood level of the drug, and/or administration of an antagonist.

III. Tolerance

Tolerance is a state of adaptation in which exposure to a drug induces changes that result in a diminution of one or more of the drug's effects over time. Most specialists in pain medicine and addiction medicine agree that patients treated with prolonged opioid therapy usually do develop physical dependence and sometimes develop tolerance, but do not usually develop addictive disorders.

Addiction is a primary chronic disease and exposure to opioid medications is only one of the etiologic factors for its development. Therefore, good clinical judgment must be used in determining whether the pattern of behaviors signals the presence of addiction or reflects a different issue.

Drug overdose has become the leading cause of injury death in the United States. More than half of those deaths involve prescription drugs, specifically opioids. A key component of addressing this national epidemic is improving prescriber practices. According to the National Institute on Drug Abuse, over 2.5 million people receive treatment each year at a qualified drug rehab facility. And although the world of addiction treatment is filled with caring, expert professionals who have dedicated their lives to helping others, there are unfortunately, a number of businesses within the industry that over-promise in terms of the results offered, or flat out lie about the effectiveness of their programs.

Allegations of fraud and other criminal practices are impacting care and prompting lawmakers to consider a plan to properly license and regulate substance abuse treatment facilities. Some clinics diagnose people with addictions they don't have, so they can increase client rolls. The clinics recruit mentally ill residents from group homes to attend therapy sessions. They attract patients from the street through incentives of cash, food and cigarettes, and have them sign in for days they do not attend sessions. One clinic billed for clients who could not have attended sessions, either because they were in jail or dead.

Eight people have been indicted for allegedly participating in a scheme that submitted more than $50 million in fraudulent bills to a California state program for alcohol and drug treatment services for high school and middle school students who, in many instances, were not provided or were provided to students who did not have substance abuse problems. Kickbacks for patient referrals for addiction treatment cost payers considerable sums of money.

Fraud in health care is just like in any other industry: Fraudsters with the means and opportunity take full advantage to unjustly profit. Health care crooks inside and outside the industry include patients, payers, employers, vendors and suppliers, and providers, including pharmacists.

When addicts want to get free of their addiction, the most common path, at least for those who can afford it, is a brief chemical detox followed by a 28-day inpatient rehab. In South Florida, rehab is often followed by a much longer stint living in a halfway house (typically a low-rent apartment) with other recovering addicts. People staying in those "sober living" homes are often encouraged to get additional support from outpatient programs that offer one-on-one counseling, group therapy, and 12-step programs. Stories abound in Delray Beach of halfway house owners charging insurance companies thousands of dollars a month for simple urine tests, collecting illegal referral fees from rehab programs, and even finding ways to get addicts drugs in hopes that they will relapse.

Health care consumers need to identify these health care fraudsters and report them to attempt to salvage the health care system. People need to remember that he/she could receive a monetary reward for being a whistle blower.

Whistle blowers are people who expose unethical or illegal wrongdoing within companies by reporting it internally to superiors or externally to the media, government authorities, or specialized attorneys. They can be either current or past employees (insiders), or outside individuals who are familiar with the unlawful conduct, and are not required to be U.S. citizens. If you properly report Medicare fraud, you may be entitled to a significant whistleblower reward.

12. Medical Laboratory Fraud

Medical laboratories are a prime target for Medicare and Medicaid fraud. In October 2015, California-based Millennium Health paid $256 million to settle the quit am allegations leveled against it. The company was accused of paying kickbacks to doctors and billing the government for unnecessary testing, including unwarranted genetic testing. One of the most widely publicized clinical lab fraud cases in U.S. history saw almost 40 healthcare providers pleading guilty to participation in a bribery scheme. According to allegations, hundreds of doctors helped defraud $100 million from healthcare programs by accepting kickbacks in exchange for patient referrals to a particular lab.

According to allegations in the criminal complaint filed a managing member of Healthcare Marketing Florida LLC, paid cash kickbacks to purported medical clinics in Miami-Dade County, Florida, in exchange for DNA test samples and patient information. The manager then allegedly provided the test samples and patient information to laboratory companies for their submission of reimbursement claims to Medicare for clinical diagnostic laboratory services. Over the past 14 months, the manager has allegedly received more than $675,000 from one of the laboratory companies for the samples.

One purpose of the Anti-Kickback Statute is to protect patients from inappropriate medical referrals or recommendations by health care professionals who may be unduly influenced by financial incentives. Providing free or below-market goods or services to a physician, who is a source of referrals, or paying such a physician more than fair market value for his or her services, could constitute illegal remuneration under the anti-kickback statute. Two examples of violations which are occurring with Laboratories are unlawful specimen processing payments and unlawful registry payments.

Laboratories pay physicians, either directly or indirectly (such as through an arrangement with a marketing or other agent) to collect, process, and package patients' blood specimens (Specimen Processing Arrangements). Payments under Specimen Processing Arrangements typically are made on a per-specimen or per-patient-encounter basis and often are associated with expensive or specialized tests.

A physician group was approached by a consultant with an "opportunity" to offer, and profit from, lab tests, including advanced cardiac marker tests, from companies. As the representative explained to the physicians, his organization would help the physicians set up and run a lab in which the physicians would own a 40% minority share. Supposedly, the lab would have been based in a small local hospital which would perform the billing. The purpose of the minority ownership was to conceal the fact that physician-owned laboratories are illegal and unethical.

The reason for billing through the local hospital was because many of the insurance companies have caught on to the fact that laboratory companies like HDL and True Health have been charging outrageous amounts for thousands of dollars' worth of unnecessary tests for their patients. But the insurance companies haven't yet caught on that the billing for these tests are now coming from small, previously reputable hospitals. The consultant even told the group of doctors that the scheme would probably last only a few years before the insurance companies caught on, but by that time the physician group and their partners would already have made a tidy profit.

Another hotspot of laboratory scams is toxicology testing. Now it is often the case that it is reasonable to require regular drug testing as a condition of receiving an opiate medication. Drug screening emerged a decade ago when pain doctors ordered tests for chronic pain patients as a precaution to protect against overprescribing charges, but said a second wave of claims has been from a profit seeking-period. Fraud experts have said drug screening has become a "money spigot,"

Urine drug testing (UDT) is an important component of the treatment plan for patients who are prescribed opioids for chronic pain. While there is not enough information so far to support a specific testing protocol for patient-centered clinical urine drug testing, experts in the fields of pain and addiction and pharmacology have developed recommendations for the use of UDT as an initial assessment and for ongoing monitoring in this population. The question of whom to test is made easier by having a uniform practice policy either in a pain or primary practice that would help reduce individual stigma. Any risk of patient profiling based on racial, cultural, or other physical appearances is eliminated. Careful explanation of the purpose of testing normally allays patient concerns.

UDT must be done routinely as part of an overall best practice program in order to prescribe chronic opioid therapy. This program may include risk stratification; baseline and periodic UDT; behavioral monitoring; and prescription monitoring programs as the best available tools to monitor chronic opioid compliance. Evidence suggests that predictors of aberrant behavior are not completely reliable, however, and that a substantial number of individuals using illicit substances will be missed if clinicians restrict urine testing to those they deem to be at high risk. Thus, UDT may be a valuable tool for low-risk patients on chronic opioid therapy, as well.

A drug test is a technical analysis of a biological specimen, for example, urine, hair, blood, breath, sweat, or oral fluid/saliva to determine the presence or absence of specified parent drugs or their metabolites. Urine analysis is primarily used because of its low cost. Urine drug testing is one of the most common testing methods used.

The rationale for performing UDT will depend on the clinical question(s) to be answered; for example, to assist in medication adherence, seeking an initial diagnosis of drug misuse or addiction, as an adjunct to self-report of drug history, to encourage or reinforce healthy behavioral change, or as a requirement of continued treatment. Doctors frequently order patients to take urine drug tests to safe-guard against prescription pain-pill abuse but federal investigators and Medicare say these routine tests designed to ensure patients properly use opioid drugs have led to questionable billing practices by some for-profit labs, doctors, and addiction-treatment centers. Urine tests can show doctors, whether their patients are taking extra pain drugs and whether they are taking their prescribed drugs.

Patients may need urine drug screening tests for a variety of reasons including monitoring of their pain medication regimen or simply as a screening tool to look for the presence of drugs. It's important to understand the types of drug screens and why one would need them prior to investigating any issues involving these tests. There is often a legitimate need for such drug tests, to determine whether an addict has relapsed or to ensure that patients prescribed painkillers are taking them rather than selling them.

There are two types of urine drug testing procedures: qualitative and quantitative. Qualitative drug screens are testing for the presence or absence of a particular drug. Quantitative drug screens are testing for how much of that substance is present. In 20 years', the number of prescriptions written for pharmaceutical drugs in the U.S. has climbed abruptly; more than six-fold, which has consequently, driven up demand for urine drug testing services by doctors trying to monitor their patients' drug intake habits.

With this explosion in the urine drug testing industry has come a wave of fraud and corruption allegations. In 2011, the average number of older Americans misusing or dependent on prescription pain relievers grew to about 336,000, up from 132,000 a decade earlier, according to the Sub-stance Abuse and Mental Health Services Administration. Medical guidelines encourage doctors who treat pain to test their patients, to make sure they are neither abusing pills nor failing to take them, possibly to sell them. Now, some pain doctors are making more from testing than from treating.

The FBI has arrested doctors for receiving kickbacks from laboratories for ordering drug testing. This behavior violated federal anti-kickback laws by giving away urine collection cups and testing strips to doctors, who say there is a growing incidence of giving workers' compensation claimants' urine drug tests even when doctors have not prescribed opioid pain medications.

Spending on the urine tests took off after Medicare cracked down on what appeared to be abusive billing for simple urine tests. Some doctors moved on to high-tech testing methods, for which billing wasn't limited. They started testing for a host of different drugs, including illegal ones that few seniors ever use and billing the federal health program for the elderly and disabled separately for each substance. Medicare's spending on 22 high-tech tests for drugs of abuse hit $445 million in 2012, up to 1, 423%% in five years. The program spent $14 million that year just on tests for angel dust. For dozens of pain doctors, Medicare payments for drug testing have eclipsed their income from treating patients. Routinely testing specimens for many different drugs is a red flag.

Safe prescribing now requires expertise in approaches that minimize the risk of unintentional overdose, drug abuse, addiction, and diversion. These approaches include urine drug testing, and while there is yet no consensus among pain specialists about the patients who should be tested and how often to test, there is broad and unqualified agreement that clinicians who treat patients with opioid drugs should be able to use urine drug testing as a tool for the assessment of drug-related behavior. There also is agreement that urine drug testing, like all tests, will yield useless information unless the indications, practicalities, and interpretation of the data are appreciated by those who order it.

Some labs encourage doctors to refer more patient specimens for drug testing by giving physicians an ownership stake or cut of test revenue, according to doctors and documents from several labs. There are some good reasons to do confirmation testing. It eliminates the risk of false-positives. The initial screening tests are very sensitive, so sometimes they incorrectly say a specimen contains evidence of drug use; the confirmation test is specific. Another reason is to measure not only whether someone is misusing drugs, but also whether they are taking therapeutic medications at the prescribed levels. There is a need for maintenance screening to determine if someone has relapsed.

There are two focal categories of urine drug testing screening: point of care followed by confirmation. Screening tests are initial, qualitative drug tests conducted to identify classes of drugs present in the urine and typically are done using immunoassay. They rely on a set threshold above which a positive result is produced and therefore, do not detect lower concentrations of a drug. Confirmatory tests are used for further analysis of a sample to confirm a positive or negative, result and typically are done using gas chromatography/mass spectrometry or high-performance liquid chromatography. Confirmatory testing can identify a specific drug. If the goal is to detect a synthetic or semisynthetic opioid, this testing should be used as immunoassays do not typically detect these opioids. Due to the possibility of false positives and the qualitative nature of screening tests, confirmatory testing is recommended to affirm positive or unexpected results and to identify the presence of a specific drug.

It is important to be sure that the drug testing occurs at a reputable and certified laboratory. A credible drug screening program will involve a two-step process. Initial (immunoassay) and confirmatory gas chromatography-mass spectrometry (GC-MS) analysis testing are the methods most commonly utilized to test for drugs. Using a combination of both tests allows a high level of sensitivity and specificity, meaning there is an extremely low chance for false positives or false negatives.

The immunoassay is performed first and is often used as a screening method. If the immunoassay is negative, no further action is required, and the results are reported as negative. If the sample is positive, an additional confirmatory GC-MS analysis is performed on a separate portion the biological sample. The more specific GC/MS is used as a confirmatory test to identify individual drug substances or metabolites and quantify the amount of the substance. Confirmatory tests, such as GC-MS should be utilized prior to reporting positive drug test results.

Many drugs stay in the system from 2 to 4 days, although the chronic use of marijuana can stay within the system for 3 to 4 weeks or even longer after the last use. Drugs with a long half-life, such as diazepam, may also stay within the system for a prolonged period of time. Drugs can be detected in hair samples up to six months. False positive drug tests are very rare in licensed, reputable laboratories. However, certain prescription medications, over-the-counter drugs, and herbal remedies can be mistaken for drugs of abuse in drug tests. For example, some decongestants might lead to a positive drug test for amphetamines.

In general, one can expect a urine test to detect drugs for the follow-ing substances: Amphetamine: 2 days, Barbiturates: two-day-3 weeks, Benzodiazepines: 3 days (therapeutic dose); 4-6 weeks (habitual use), Cocaine: four days, Ecstasy: two days, Heroin: two days, Marijuana: 2-7 days (single use); 1-2+ months (habitual use), Methamphetamine: two days, Morphine: two days, PCP: 8-14 days (single use); 30 days (chronic use). Be aware that an individual can do the following to a urine sample: dilution is the process of reducing the concentration of drug or drug metabolites in the sample. This is accomplished by adding fluid to the sample, and some sites online may recommend it. However, drug testing laboratories all routinely test samples to detect dilution.

One method of diluting the sample involves adding liquid to urine. However, the temperature of the urine is measured by drug tests, and diluted urine is easily detected. Substitution is a method that involves substituting your urine with that of another person's or a synthetic sample. There are many companies that sell devices for urine substitution over the Internet, as well as companies that sell synthetic urine. Point of Care cups (POC) are enzyme mediated immunoassay (EIA) devices. These are cups with strips that change color and are similar to urine pregnancy tests. They are the least expensive, and least accurate, of all the urine monitoring tools. To use these, the doctor needs no special equipment or training.

In 2009, the American Pain Society and the American Academy of Pain Medicine convened an expert panel that developed Clinical Guidelines for the Use of Chronic Opioid Therapy in Chronic Noncancerous Pain. The panel concluded that UDT has a central role in monitoring patients receiving chronic opioid therapy to avoid its potential harms. Specifically, the panel recommended that UDT should be used periodically in all treated patients who are at high risk for abuse or diversion, and that UDT should also be considered even for patients who do not have known risk factors in order to confirm adherence to the chronic opioid therapy plan of care.

In the panel's opinion, UDT should be considered for all patients, including those without apparent elevated risk, as part of the protocol of practices, especially when controlled substances, such as opioids, are pre-scribed. The literature is clear that when aberrant behavior alone is used as a trigger for UDT, a significant proportion of patients who would benefit from this technology will be missed. Therefore, a consistent clinical approach in performing UDT will optimize the use of this technology for both patient and practitioner alike.

Provider fraud may occur with respect to drug testing. A Dallas health care provider has faced allegations that it paid millions in kickbacks to physicians and others for patient referrals. The number of federal health care kickback cases is spreading nationwide. The Justice Department has targeted labs, pharmacies, physicians, chiropractors and hospitals in recent years and company-paid sales brokers to find medical providers willing to engage in the illegal kickback scheme, the lawsuit said. The kickbacks were disguised as payment for administrative, marketing or consulting services.

A minority of drug screening laboratories received nearly $100 mil-lion from Oklahoma's Medicaid program over the last five years, prompting an investigation from state officials. Between 2011 and 2014, Oklahoma's annual reimbursement to urine testing laboratories increased more than 700 percent, from $3.7 million to $32 million, and threatened to drain the state's healthcare budget. The labs often billed for medically unnecessary tests, or billed for more expensive quantitative panel tests that cost as much as $800, according to the Oklahoma Health Care Authority. Several labs also engaged in kickback schemes, compensating physicians in exchange for referrals.

A physicians group has agreed to pay $7.4 million to the federal government to resolve allegations that it violated the False Claims Act by performing medically unnecessary drug screen procedures, the U.S. Department of Justice said Wednesday. The settlement relates to the business' use of tests that identify and count particles of illicit drugs in patients' urine. The DOJ said the quantitative drug tests, which are very specific and expensive, are appropriate only if there is reason to doubt the more general and cheaper qualitative drug test screens. However, the DOJ said regardless of results of the less-expensive test, Coastal performed and billed all patients for the quantitative drug tests.

A laboratory in California allegedly billed Medicare, Medicaid and other federal health care programs for medically unnecessary urine drug and genetic testing, and for providing free items to physicians who agreed to refer expensive laboratory testing business to this laboratory. Another physician group was approached by a laboratory sales consultant with an opportunity to offer, And profit from, lab tests. As the representative explained to the physicians, his organization would help the physicians set up and run a lab in which the physicians would own a 40% minority share.

Presumably the lab would have been based in a small local hospital which would perform the billing. The purpose of the minority ownership was to conceal the fact that physician-owned laboratories are illegal and unethical. The reason for billing through the local hospital was because many of the insurance companies have caught on to the fact that laboratory companies have been charging despicable amounts for unnecessary tests for their patients. However, few insurance companies haven't discovered that the billings for these tests are now coming from small, previously reputable hospitals.

Patients need to be aware of possible fraudulent laboratory practices and if these practices are in question, the patient should notify his/her or her insurance carrier.

Health care consumers need to identify these health care fraudsters and report them to attempt to salvage the health care system. People need to remember that he/she could receive a monetary reward for being a whistle blower.

Whistle blowers are people who expose unethical or illegal wrongdoing within companies by reporting it internally to superiors or externally to the media, government authorities, or specialized attorneys. They can be either current or past employees (insiders), or

outside individuals who are familiar with the unlawful conduct, and are not required to be U.S. citizens. If you properly report Medicare fraud, you may be entitled to a significant whistleblower reward.

13. Pharmacy Fraud

Pharmacy is the science and technique of preparing and dispensing drugs. It is a health profession that links health sciences with chemical sciences and aims to ensure the safe and effective use of pharmaceutical drugs. A pharmacist is another individual in health care who could scam you. Prescription-drug abuse causes many more problems and is much more common than the common "street" drugs such as heroin and cocaine. Prescription-drug abuse causes many deaths every day through mixing various medications or using the drugs for recreation when they were not medically prescribed to the individual.

Because of the high desire of illegal prescription drugs, this makes medications very attractive for criminals. Drug diversion is where a prescription drug is taken out of the normal chain of commerce and diverted for sale or use in some illegal activity. Often these diverted drugs are billed to Medicaid before they are stolen. One area of concern is prescription shorting. This is where a fraudulent pharmacy routinely dispenses prescriptions a few pills short. In a large prescription, the pharmacist hopes the beneficiary will not notice.

A fraudulent pharmacy may fill a partial month's drug supply and ask the beneficiary to return for the rest. The pharmacist then bills Medicaid twice in one month for the full amount. Criminal enterprises posing as pharmacies are billing Medicare, Medicaid and private insurers for fake prescriptions and bilking health care out of millions of dollars. Criminals may use a legitimate address to establish a fake pharmacy business. Using stolen or otherwise stolen doctor ID and patient insurance ID numbers, scammers write fraudulent prescriptions for expensive drugs that were never actually prescribed or dispensed. They submit these fake prescriptions for reimbursement to insurers. Criminals quickly make large amounts of money, then close up and open up a new scam somewhere else.

Evidence presented at a six-week jury trial concluding in August 2012 showed between 2006 and 2011, several pharmacies billed Medicare and Medicaid more than $57 million. At least 25 percent of those billings were for drugs that were either medically unnecessary never dispensed. The pharmacies operated on a business model that paid kickbacks to physicians in exchange for writing prescriptions for expensive medications. The affiliated doctors would also write prescriptions for controlled substances, without regard to medical necessity, which would be filled at the pharmacies and distributed to paid "patients" and patient recruiters. The expensive, non-controlled medications would be billed but not dispensed.

A pharmacist was making free money by billing expensive false prescription claims to unsuspecting payers. When he needed some extra cash, he would invent a disease scenario for an existing patient; submit a claim for a false prescription to a payer via computer. Some pharmacies recycle and reuse pills that were returned from nursing homes to resell or charge the whole price for a prescription even though it was only partially filled for the customer. In California, a physician and pharmacist, plus 3 other individuals, were charged for allegedly participating in bribes and kickbacks to physicians in exchange for prescribing expensive equipment and compounded pain creams that were medically unnecessary.

A pharmacy owner admitted that between October 2012 and September 2013, the pharmacy submitted nearly $1.6 million in fraudulent claims to Medicare for prescription drugs that were not prescribed by physicians. A multimillion-dollar fraud scheme was discovered, which involved prescription compounding pharmacies. Each of the men was charged with conspiracy to commit health care fraud and wire fraud, and some were charged with money laundering as well. According to the indictment, the co-conspirators allegedly used several Miami area pharmacies to submit false and fraudulent reimbursement claims for prescription compounded medications to private insurance firms, Medicare, and Tricare between October 2012 and December 2015.

The report alleges the pharmacies submitted about $633 million in claims for prescription compounded medications and received about $157 million in reimbursement based on those claims. The indictment also says the conspirators allegedly used shell companies to transfer and disburse the money and to hide their involvement in the scheme.

Pharmacy fraud has become a rampant problem spreading from Miami across much of Florida, as drug traffickers conspire with doctors and sometimes patients to cheat the Medicare system, a federal investigator told the Senate Committee on Aging on Wednesday.

A report estimated that approximately 2,600 retail drugstores, or 4% of all U.S. pharmacies participating in Medicare, submitted suspicious or excessive billings to the federal government. The report also stated that 2,637 pharmacies submitted suspect billings for about $5.6 billion in 2009. In the context of all pharmacies operating throughout the country, chain stores were involved in 1% of the alleged fraudulent practices, and 11% of all independents submitted false or inflated claims for payment. Another pharmacy group is accused of masterminding a complex insurance fraud scheme of recruiting doctors and pharmacists to prescribe unnecessary treatment for workers' compensation insurance patients.

Two other pharmacists were accused of conspiring with two individuals by selling more than $1 million in compound creams that were not FDA approved nor have known medical benefits. "These individuals and their co-conspirators played with patients' lives, buying and selling them for profit without regard to patient safety," said a prosecutor. "Patients have the right to expect treatment decisions by health care professionals are based on medical need and not unadulterated greed. The magnitude of this alleged crime is an affront to ethical medical professionals."

These co-conspirators are accused of making oral and written agreements with doctors across the state paying them each time they prescribed a compound cream or oral medication or ordered a urine drug test. The doctors or the companies connected to them are accused of labeling the payments "marketing expenses" in an attempt to conceal the kickbacks. The co-conspirators were accused of rewarding doctors who provided a higher volume by paying for office technicians. The co-conspirators were also accused of purchasing repackaged oral pain medications from two companies: NuCare Pharmaceuticals in Orange and A-S Medication Solutions in Costa Mesa. Using their company Monarch Medical Group as a cover, the co-conspirators are accused of repackaging meds sent directly to the physicians involved in the scam.

As the doctors dispensed the medication, the bar code on the packaging was scanned, notifying the co-conspirators. They are accused of billing workers' compensation insurance carriers without disclosing the wholesale cost or the fact they had purchased the medication on behalf of the physicians who ultimately prescribed it. Once the co-conspirators received the payment, they are accused of splitting the profits with the prescribing physician based upon a pre-arranged agreement.

Five doctors alone prescribed more than 500,000 doses of oxycodone, which had a street value of $10 million; 2 million doses of hydrocodone; more than 2 million doses of alprazolam (Xanax); and more than 1,000 L of codeine-based cough syrup over a 21-month period. The suspects are charged with running a criminal operation complete with bribery, money laundering, kickbacks, and guns that bilked Medicare of more than $21.5 million. Health care fraud charges were filed against 32 of the defendants; three are charged with money laundering, and three are also charged with being felons in possession of firearms.

Two Irvine pharmacists were accused of conspiring by selling more than $1 million in compound creams that were not federally approved nor have any known medical benefits. More than 13,000 patients and at least 27 insurance carriers statewide were victims in the scheme, which the Orange County District Attorney's office says took place between 2011 to 2015 and involved billing for unnecessary creams, tests, and treatments to maximize profits. According to prosecutors, these individuals worked with pharmacists to manufacture a variety of creams with unknown effects that were not FDA approved. After purchasing assorted creams for between $15 and $40 per tube, the products were then billed to patients' workers' compensation insurance carriers for between $250 and $700 dollars per tube. Physicians were allegedly invited to participate in the scheme by offering a flat $50 rate or a share in the profits.

Federal prosecutors have opened investigations in at least four states into compounding pharmacies that allegedly issued false claims to a U.S. military health insurance program in violation of the federal False Claims Act. In Florida, four pharmacies previously agreed to pay a total of $12.8 million in civil settlements that they allegedly falsely billed the military insurance program Tricare.

Two of the pharmacies employed people who allegedly paid doctors to write prescriptions for Tricare patients, even if the doctors hadn't met the patients, prosecutors said. Another pharmacy allegedly gave commissions to marketers who promoted their drugs. Some pharmacies charged Tricare from $10,000 to $40,000 for a month of compounded medicines.

Compounding pharmacies alter the dosage or form of a drug from what's commercially available. "A growing number of people and animals have unique health needs that off-the-shelf, one-size-fits-all prescription medicines cannot meet. Some valuable medications are available only by compounding. In 2014, Tricare spent about $500 million on compounded drugs. In 2015 it has spent an estimated $1.75 billion.

Health care consumers need to identify these health care fraudsters and report them to attempt to salvage the health care system. People need to remember that he/she could receive a monetary reward for being a whistle blower.

Whistle blowers are people who expose unethical or illegal wrongdoing within companies by reporting it internally to superiors or externally to the media, government authorities, or specialized attorneys. They can be either current or past employees (insiders), or outside individuals who are familiar with the unlawful conduct, and are not required to be U.S. citizens. If you properly report Medicare fraud, you may be entitled to a significant whistleblower reward.

14. Compound Drug Fraud

Topical medications can be fraudulent as well the other medications previously mentioned. The fastest-growing categories of compounded drugs are topical creams and gels, often used for pain. Pain relievers can be applied directly to your skin. These topical pain relievers are a noninvasive and convenient method for delivering pain-relieving medications. This is especially important and beneficial if you are not able to take medications by mouth. Topical pain relievers include complementary and alternative medications as well as conventional medications. Topical forms of analgesics, or pain relievers, have been used through-out human history.

The use of ointments for medicinal purposes is mentioned in the Bible. The purpose of a topical analgesic is to transmit a medication through your skin into your body. The amount of drug that actually gets through your skin is determined by the amount of pressure applied as you rub it over your skin, the area of your skin covered by the drug, the thickness of your skin and the way in which the drug is dissolved, and the use of dressings over your skin. Analgesics are available in ointments, creams, and gels. They also may be placed in patches that may be applied to your skin.

The advantage of topical analgesics is that they can be placed on the skin over the site of your pain. When compared to oral medications, you will have a lower blood level of the drug and will have fewer side effects and fewer drug interactions. There are different types of topical pain relievers. Ointments are semisolid preparations that melt at body temperature and spread easily. Ointments are not routinely used for the practice of pain medicine unless the ointment is specially compounded by a pharmacy.

Ointments are defined in three categories based on your skin penetration. One type of ointment does not penetrate beyond the external layer of your skin called the epidermis. Ointments of this class can be used in the treatment of sunburn. A second type of ointment penetrates to the internal layer of your skin called the dermis. The third type of ointment actually goes through your skin to the nerves and ligaments and in some instances into your bloodstream. The latter two types of ointments are frequently used in pain management.

Substances applied on your skin can evaporate. You do not want your analgesic drug evaporating from your skin. Your pharmacist will add substances such as glycerin to the ointment to keep this evaporation from happening. Ointments can be prepared by your pharmacist or purchased over the counter or by prescription. Some ointment preparations will contain absorption enhancers. Absorption enhancers make it easier for the drug to be absorbed through your skin. Azone and DMSO can both enhance the absorption of ointments through your skin. Ointments should be packaged in tubes.

Creams are opaque, thick, liquid substances that consist of medications dissolved in a cream base that usually vanishes through the skin. They are less of a liquid consistency than ointments. Gels are a drug-delivery system that usually contain penetration enhancers and are usually used for administering anti-inflammatory medications. The anti-inflammatory medication must be absorbed through your skin to provide you with pain relief. Gels are useful treatment methods if you have arthritic and/or muscle pain. Gels usually are thicker than creams or ointments and are usually clear, unlike creams and ointments.

The concentration of medication in gels is usually no greater than 2 percent. For example, lidocaine, which is a numbing medicine for the control of pain, is dispensed as a 2 percent gel. However, the cream is available in a 5 percent concentration. This is because medications are usually absorbed through the skin better if used in gel form. Gels usually have clarity and sparkle. They maintain their thickness even with an elevated body temperature. Some gels have been developed that may be given nasally. Some drugs are absorbed well through your nose than through your skin. Gels are usually dispensed into tubes or squeeze bottles.

Another delivery system for analgesics is a transdermal patch, which contains medication that is transmitted directly through your skin. A patch containing a medication is placed on your skin and remains there for a specified time so that the drug within the patch can be delivered through your skin to your bloodstream. Local anesthetics such as lidocaine, capsaicin cream, and fentanyl (a potent opioid medication), are some of the medicines that can be delivered through your skin using a transdermal drug delivery system.

Another topical medication used to prevent pain is EMLA cream. This cream is dispensed only by prescription. It is used as a numbing agent more than it is used for reducing pain. This is a cream consisting of lidocaine and prilocaine, which are both numbing agents. This local anesthetic combination is packaged in tubes. An EMLA cellulose disc can be applied over your painful area. The purpose of EMLA is to provide pain relief over the painful area of your skin. It is used in children to reduce the pain of starting intravenous lines. Some pain-management doctors advocate its use to decrease the pain associated with reflex sympathetic dystrophy or the pain associated with shingles. This cream should be placed on an intact skin area.

The EMLA should be applied under a bandage for at least 60 minutes to provide relief over the painful area of your skin. This cream is not recommended if you have an allergy to lidocaine or prilocaine. If you have the blood disorder called methemoglobinemia, you should not use this cream. You should not exceed the recommended dose prescribed by your physician.

Nonsteroidal anti-inflammatory agents (NSAIDS) may be compounded into creams by your pharmacist. These creams should not be used more than three times a day. Side effects with the nonsteroidal anti-inflammatory creams are the same as with the NSAIDs taken by mouth. However, the side effects of the topical NSAIDS are less than the oral NSAIDS. The side effects of any NSAID can include stomach upset and allergic reactions. If the dose is high enough, it could affect both your liver and kidneys. These NSAIDs can be very effective for the management of your pain when applied over your skin.

The transdermal fentanyl patch system has become popular since it was introduced in the 1980s. This strong opioid medication was used initially for cancer pain management and then for noncancerous, chronic pain management. Fentanyl is able to penetrate your skin easily. Fentanyl is 75 times more potent than morphine. It produces fewer histamine releases from cells in your bloodstream and causes less itching than morphine. The fentanyl patch is primarily used for chronic or cancer-related pain.

When the fentanyl patch is placed on your skin, the fentanyl diffuses through the holes in the release membrane to the surface of your skin. It then goes to the outer layer of your skin and is deposited in a storage area. From the storage area, it is gradually absorbed into your blood-stream. This is the reason that it takes at least an hour before the fentanyl has begun to enter your bloodstream.

You will probably not notice any pain-relieving effects from this drug-delivery system for about six hours. The patch is usually removed every three days. After the patch is removed, you will still have some drug that remains within the storage area under your skin. If you remove the patch and do not replace it, you will still receive fentanyl for hours after the patch has been removed.

The Lidoderm transdermal drug-delivery system exerts a significant amount of its pain-relieving effects by releasing a small amount of lidocaine into your bloodstream. Lidocaine is a local anesthetic. The patch does not cause numbness over your skin but does give you some degree of pain relief below the patch. There also is an effect upon the nerves under your skin that are transmitting pain. This patch is used for the treatment of shingles. The Lidoderm patch contains 5 percent lidocaine. The lidocaine essentially does not reach your bloodstream like fentanyl.

The lidocaine penetrates your skin just enough to reach the nerve endings that are transmitting your pain. As a result, there are minimal side effects from the use of this patch other than from the adhesive layer of the patch. The amount of the lidocaine that is absorbed from the Lidoderm is related to the length of application over your skin. The patch should be used within 12 hours over your painful area and then removed for 12 hours. If an irritation or a burning sensation occurs around the adhesive aspect of the patch, you should discontinue use of the patch. None of the patches mentioned throughout this chapter should ever be reused.

Clonidine is another transdermal medication (Catepress). This patch is applied weekly to one area of your skin. The clonidine patch inhibits the release of norepinephrine, which is a pain transmitter. The clonidine patch also is used in the treatment of hypertension. If you have neuropathic (nerve injury) pain or reflex sympathetic dystrophy, the clonidine patch may provide you with significant pain relief. It also can be successfully used if you have pain following shingles.

Some compounding pharmacies are preparing compounded pain creams and ointments that contain a combination of multiple potent medications. Many include drugs that can cause central nervous system depression or cardiac effects such as ketamine, baclofen, cyclobenzaprine, lidocaine, tricyclic antidepressants, gabapentin, clonidine, and nifedipine. Most of these drugs have not been US Food and Drug Administration (FDA)-approved for topical use.

Southern California doctors were bribed to prescribe a pain-relief concoction as part of a $25 million workers' compensation scam.

Prosecutors contend that Kareem Ahmed hired pharmacists to produce a pain-relief cream, gave kickbacks to doctors and chiropractors to prescribe it to workers' compensation patients, and conspired to submit phony claims.

Prosecutors alleged insurance fraud and conspiracy in a 44-count indictment, with crimes occurring from Oct. 1, 2009, through Jan. 31, 2013. Kickbacks to individuals were as high as $8 million over multiple years, the indictment said. It's a robocall, and it tells you that you have been selected to receive free pain relief cream. All you have to do is follow the prompts and arranges for delivery.

Sometimes a patient will receive a robocall to promote a topical pain cream. "In an attempt to stop the growing use and abuse of prescription narcotic pain pills, America's national health-care providers are now authorized to provide a new experimental pain relief compound to anyone suffering from physical pain or discomfort," the robocall says. "This compound cream is directly applied to the pain-related areas," it continues. "It is non-narcotic and extremely effective. This new pain relief compound is provided to you by your insurance carrier with no out-of-pocket expense to you, and your pain-relief cream can be shipped immediately."

The Food and Drug Administration (FDA) is warning five firms, Triangle Compounding Pharmacy, University Pharmacy, Custom Scripts Pharmacy, Hal's Compounding Pharmacy, and New England Compounding Center, to stop compounding and distributing standardized versions of topical anesthetic creams, which are marketed for general distribution rather than responding to the unique medical needs of individual patients. Firms that do not resolve violations in FDA warning letters risk enforcement such as injunctions against continuing violations and seizure of illegal products.

The FDA is concerned about the serious public health risks related to compounded topical anesthetic creams. Exposure to high concentrations of local anesthetics, like those in compounded topical anesthetic creams, can cause grave reactions, including seizures and irregular heartbeats. Two deaths have been connected to compounded topical anesthetic creams made by Triangle Compounding Pharmacy and University Pharmacy, two of the five pharmacies receiving warning letters. Similar topical anesthetic creams are compounded by the other firms, and today's action serves as a general warning to firms that produce standardized versions of these creams.

Some of the prescriptions may not have been medically necessary or even dispensed at all, notes the report, which also details recent fraud cases brought by U.S. attorneys in several states. Use among Medicare beneficiaries and federal employees in workers' compensation insurance plans has recently soared.

In Florida, federal prosecutors unsealed an indictment against a doctor who allegedly was given kickbacks, including a BMW for sending prescriptions to a particular pharmacy, which then billed Tricare, Medicare and other government health programs for compounded creams. Prices ranged from about $900 to $21,000 for a one-month supply.

Two pharmacies paid kickbacks to prescribing physicians in the form of "research fees." For researching pain creams. Another Florida pharmacy disguised $70,000 in kickbacks as speaker's fees for an Indiana physician. Marketing firms that steered Tricare beneficiaries to compounding pharmacies received kickbacks as well, prosecutors said.

The United States alleges that four physicians had an incentive to refer prescriptions to their pharmacy, as steering costly prescriptions to the pharmacy Topical Specialists resulted in lucrative revenue streams for the doctors. The United States contends that these four physicians wrote hundreds of prescriptions for pain and scar creams. After speaking with patients, the government contends that these prescriptions were often not used by patients, despite the tremendous cost for the government.

While the pharmacies billed the federal government tens of thousands of dollars for these creams, the cost to actually compound them was often 4-5% of the submitted cost. Records reviewed by the government showed that the pharmacy was making up to 90% profit for each cream submitted to the Tricare health insurance program. This profit was then disbursed to the doctors who wrote the prescriptions.

In some cases, the four physicians recruited other doctors to write prescriptions – and shared their revenue with them. The government alleges that in some cases, the doctors who wrote prescriptions to Topical Specialists and WELL Health received up to 40% of the reimbursement. All four physicians received hundreds of thousands of dollars in reimbursements.

Topical cream manufacturers have fallen under scrutiny of the law for incentivizing prescribers to utilize these products. In Southern California, the Orange County grand jury has indicted 15 people involved with defrauding over $100 million from insurance companies. "We believe there were thousands of prescriptions being written and thousands being filled by multiple pharmacies in Orange County," and there were "huge markups billed to insurance companies," Workers' compensation insurers were billed in "the $1,500 to $3,000 range" for creams that had a wholesale cost of about $70.

The FDA keeps watch over topical medication scams.

Health care consumers need to identify these health care fraudsters and report them to attempt to salvage the health care system. People need to remember that he/she could receive a monetary reward for being a whistle blower. Whistle blowers are people who expose unethical or illegal wrongdoing within companies by reporting it internally to superiors or externally to the media, government authorities, or specialized attorneys. They can be either current or past employees (insiders), or outside individuals who are familiar with the unlawful conduct, and are not

15. Alternative Medicine Fraud

Wikipedia describes alternative medicine as health care that includes practices claimed to have the healing effects of medicine but, which are disproven, unproven, impossible to prove, or are excessively harmful in relation to their effect; and where the scientific consensus is that the therapy does not, or cannot, work because the known laws of nature are violated by its basic claims; or where it is considered so much worse than conventional treatment that it would be unethical to offer as treatment.

The term "alternative medicine" encompasses a wide array of health care practices, products, and therapies that are distinct from practices, products, and therapies used in conventional medicine. Examples of alternative medicine include homeopathic, traditional Chinese, and Ayurvedic medicine. Alternative medicine may be very effective in decreasing your pain. Many conventional medicine pain practices include alternative medicine clinicians as part of their multidisciplinary treatment. For example, practices include alternative medicine clinicians as part of their multidisciplinary treatment. For example, acupuncture may be offered in some pain practices. "Conventional medicine" is practiced by medical doctors (M.D.) or doctors of osteopathy (D.O.).

There are two main categories of frauds in alternative medicine. One category consists of illegitimate therapies that are emulations of poisonous orthodox medicine, such as the use of radiation. The other category of alternative medicine frauds is much more disturbing. This latter category is heavily influenced by dark religions. Due to the religious undertones, many of the involved lost refer to themselves as being "spiritual."

Conventional medicine includes methods practiced by allied health-care professionals such as physical therapists, occupational therapists, psychologists, and registered nurses. Other terms for conventional medicine include allopathic medicine, mainstream medicine, and orthodox medicine. There are two main categories of frauds in alternative medicine. One category consists of illegitimate therapies that are emulations of poisonous orthodox medicine, such as the use of radiation. The other category of alternative medicine frauds is much more disturbing. This latter category is heavily influenced by dark religions.

In general, health fraud drug products are articles of unproven effectiveness that claim to treat disease or improve health. In addition to wasting billions of consumers' dollars each year, health scams can lead patients to delay proper treatment and cause serious and even fatal injuries. The FDA is very concerned about these fraud products, and removing these products from the market remains one of the Agency's top priorities.

The National Institute of Health (NIH) is reviewing alternative therapies and is confirming efficacy and safety in some areas. Complementary and alternative medicines, unlike many conventional medicine therapies, are designed to help you develop control over your health. If you are going to use any of these methods, you are encouraged to learn the side effects of some of these medicines as well as learn about drug interactions with conventional medications.

All plants have different amounts of substances in them. A true dose of an alternative medication in a pill is unknown in many instances. You should look carefully at the label before taking one of these substances and not take more than the label recommends. The overall drug interactions of herbal substances have not been established because they are not required to be studied by the FDA.

Some health plans have now announced their intention to incorporate payment for some alternative medicine practices into their insurance coverage. Some managed care corporations have revealed their intentions to include alternative medicine practices for payment. Some state governments are considering legislation pertaining to the practice of alternative medicine by health-care professionals.

Healthcare fraud remains a broad regulatory category that enforcement authorities can use against the manufacturer or distributor of a healthcare product that raises questions in the minds of officials. Even though the FDA has indicated greater tolerance for complementary and alternative medicine products, by issuing its permissive draft guidance on low-risk, general wellness products. The FDA maintains a web page on Alternative Medicine Fraud.

There are risks and benefits that you should be aware of when using alternative medications and therapies to manage your pain. In addition, the alternative medications you take could react with the prescription medications your doctor has given you and cause you even more problems. For example, high doses of vitamin E can decrease your blood's ability to form a blood clot.

In 1994, Congress passed the Dietary Supplement Health and Education Act. In passing this act, Congress recognized that many individuals believed that dietary supplements offered health benefits. The bill gave dietary supplement manufacturers freedom to produce more products and to provide information about their products' health benefits. The Food and Drug Administration (FDA), on the other hand, is responsible for overseeing any claims by the dietary supplement The FDA monitors manufacturers to the truthfulness of their claims.

The Federal Trade Commission regulates the advertising of all of the dietary supplements. You should be aware that the quality control standards for natural substances are a problem within this industry. Some of the manufacturers of these products will not have the amount of substance in the natural medication as stated on the container label. The overall drug interactions of herbal substances have not been established because they are not required to be studied by the FDA. You must do your own research to determine whether the natural substance that you are taking has an accurate dosage as stated on the container label for the product.

For example, if you want acupuncture, you should inquire if there are state requirements for the practice of acupuncture. Someone who is not trained could cause you harm. The NIH does award grants for the study of research in complementary as well as alternative medicines. Clinical trials are being done throughout the United States with respect to complementary and alternative medicines. You may want to participate in one of these trials.

Study trials with respect to herbal medicines are an important part of the medical research process. The results from clinical trials can define better ways to treat your painful conditions. A clinical trial is a research study in which a therapy is tested on individuals like you to ensure that the medicine being tested is safe and effective. Always remember that clinical trials have risks. Before participating in a clinical trial, discuss this trial with your primary-care physician. To find out about ongoing clinical trials, for example, studies on arthritis and neurological disorders go to www.nccam.nih.gov.

You also may want to access the National Library of Medicine online (www.pubmed.com.). Complementary medicine on PubMed is available that contains citations to articles on recently published research. You may want to see a homeopathic or naturopathic specialist. Homeopathic specialists prescribe dilutions of natural substances from plants, minerals, and animals. Homeopathy has been around for more than 200 years.

It is important to know that the U.S. Food and Drug Administration recognizes homeopathic remedies as official drugs and regulates their manufacture. This is unlike the herbs used for medicinal use. Conventional physicians in Europe use homeopathy qualities of medicine frequently. In Britain, homeopathy is a part of the national health system.

The basic principles of homeopathy are that a disease can be destroyed and removed by a type of medicine that can produce the disease in humans. In other words, a substance that in large doses would produce symptoms of a disease can be used in very minute doses to cure it. In conventional medicine, this is called the theory of antibiotics. Homeopathic practitioners adhere to the fact that the more a substance is diluted, the more potent it is. In conventional medicine, it is believed that a higher dose of the medicine will lead to a greater effect. The purpose of diluting out substances in homeopathic medicine is to avoid side effects. Homeopathic practitioners adhere to the fact that illness is different for every person. Homeopathic treatments are unique to each patient.

Homeopathic medicine emphasizes that patients are individuals and have individual signs and symptoms of an illness and should be treated only on an individual basis. The entire individual is treated, which includes the physical, psychological and spiritual portions of each person. Naturopathic medicine treats disease by using your body's natural ability to heal itself. Naturopathic practitioners invoke healing processes by using a variety of treatment options based on your particular needs. In naturopathic medicine, disease symptoms are a sign of your body's attempt to heal itself.

Dietary supplements are recommended in complimentary medicine. Dietary supplements also have unseen harms. For example, kava can cause severe and occasionally fatal liver damage; blue cohosh can cause heart failure; nutmeg can cause hallucinations; comfrey can cause hepatitis; monkshood can cause heart arrhythmias; wormwood can cause seizures; stevia leaves can decrease fertility, concentrated green tea extracts can damage the liver; bitter orange can cause heart damage, and Aristo lochia, found in Chinese herbs, can cause kidney failure and bladder cancer.

If you have developed tophi (nodules under your skin) that are painful, you may need to have these uric acid crystals removed surgically. If you have had significant destruction of one of your joints, an orthopedic surgeon may need to surgically correct any malformation that may be related to uric acid deposition in your joints and the resultant joint naturally. Naturopathic medicine gets its data from Chinese, Native American, and Greek cultures.

Reflexology is another method used in non-conventional medicine practice to decrease your pain. Reflexology relieves muscle stress and relaxes your muscles through the application of pressure on specific areas of your feet. Reflexology has been used for thousands of years in mid-eastern countries. In the early twentieth century, a doctor mapped the foot areas that related to areas of the body that affected different medical conditions. Reflexology can be used for the management of your back pain. Reflexology practitioners believe that nerve endings in the feet have inner connection throughout the spinal cord and brain to reach all areas of the body. The problem with reflexology is that it has not been scientifically studied and still remains an unproven treatment regimen for the management of your pain.

A therapeutic massage can significantly help you control your pain, especially if you have muscle spasms. Massage therapy can decrease your stress as well as decrease your headaches and pain associated with whiplash injuries. Massage therapy promotes generalized body relaxation. Massage is the application of touch to your muscles or ligaments that does not cause you to move or change position of a joint. Massage therapy can decrease your lower-back pain as well as your neck pain. It also has been effective to reduce pain associated with sciatica. Massage therapy can decrease the pain associated with tension headaches.

There are different types of massage therapy. The Swedish massage is the most common form of massage therapy in the United States. Swedish massage works on the superficial layers of the skin as well as the superficial muscles throughout your body. Swedish massage promotes relaxation and improves circulation in your superficial muscles. Another type of massage is a deep-tissue massage. This is more direct pressure on the deeper muscle layers of your body.

Deep-tissue massage is highly effective for the treatment of lower-back pain. Sports massage combines Swedish massage with deep-tissue massage. This type of massage therapy can decrease your pain following a vigorous athletic workout. It may not be a good idea to use therapeutic massage if you have certain forms of cancer, heart disease, or some infectious diseases.

Another method to help you control your pain is aromatherapy. Women have a better perception of smell than men. Therefore, women are more likely to use aromatherapy because they have better results from this method than men. Aromatherapy is reportedly effective for the treatment of muscle pain as well as pain that originates from a nerve injury. You must not use any of the aromatherapy oils if you are allergic to the herbs from which the oils were derived. If you have trouble breathing, you should not use aroma-therapy. Some aromatherapy can cause drowsiness.

Sage, rosemary, and juniper oils may increase uterine contractions if you are pregnant. You should not use these oils during pregnancy. Essential oils such as clove, cinnamon, and thyme can have anti-inflammatory proper-ties and are useful in decreasing your joint pain if you have arthritis. Aroma-therapy can be used in the following preparations: nose drops, air sprays, steam tents, candles, and drops in your bath.

Acupuncture is another popular method that can be used for pain management. Acupuncture can decrease both your pain as well as your stress. Acupuncture originated in China more than 2,000 years ago. Acupuncture is based on the belief that your health is determined by a balanced flow of vital life energy referred to as chi. Needles are inserted just under your skin to stimulate these meridians and provide you with pain relief.

It is believed that acupuncture releases the body's own chemicals that relieve pain, called endorphins and encephalin. These two chemicals are your body's natural pain-killing chemicals. Acupuncture can decrease the production as well as the distribution of substances that cause pain nerve impulses to go to the brain. Acupuncture, therefore, can decrease your need for conventional pain pills. Acupuncture has been demonstrated to decrease muscle-tension headaches.

In 1997, the National Institutes of Health endorsed acupuncture for postoperative pain, dental pain, tennis elbow, and carpal tunnel syndrome. The World Health Organization has reported that acupuncture can be useful in the treatment of migraine headaches, trigeminal neuralgia, sciatica, and arthritis.

Acupuncture also can be used to treat fibromyalgia, neck pain, and back pain. In some states, there is no licensing required to be an acupuncturist, whereas other states limit the practice to medical doctors and chiropractors. In some states, acupuncturists are considered primary health-care professionals and may see you without your doctor's referral.

Naturopaths recommend healing of the person and not the disease. Naturopathic medicinal treatments will include doses of natural substances that are much higher than those used by practitioners of homeopathic medicine. To best choose a natural product to decrease your pain, you should know which chemicals in the body produce pain. With this knowledge, you can pick the analgesic best suited to relieve your pain. If you have joint pain, for instance, you will want to use an alternative medicine that has anti-inflammatory properties.

Given that no two people are alike, if you are taking any medications and begin to take nutritional supplements you should be aware that potential drug-nutrient interactions may occur and are encouraged to consult a health-care professional before using any natural product. Combining certain prescription drugs and dietary supplements can lead to undesirable effects such as: diminished prescription-drug effectiveness, reduced supplement effectiveness and impaired drug and/or supplement absorption.

The FDA has issued a number of warning letters against companies that promoted alternative medicine products. In 2009, the FDA advised consumers not to use certain Zicam cold remedies; FDA also warned consumers against loss of smell associated with certain intranasal cold remedies containing zinc. Further research is needed.

Health care consumers need to identify these health care fraudsters and report them to attempt to salvage the health care system. People need to remember that he/she could receive a monetary reward for being a whistle blower.

Whistle blowers are people who expose unethical or illegal wrongdoing within companies by reporting it internally to superiors or externally to the media, government authorities, or specialized attorneys. They can be either current or past employees (insiders), or outside individuals who are familiar with the unlawful conduct, and are

not required to be U.S. citizens. If you properly report Medicare fraud, you may be entitled to a significant whistleblower

16. Drug Cost Fraud

When Medicare was first initiated, President George Bush assured pharmaceutical manufactures that drug pricing would continue to remain elevated. Drug prices at pharmacies in other countries are much cheaper than in the United States. Drugs in other countries can be purchased much cheaper than in the United States for the same drug.

Medical care expenditures are out of control in the United States. This is the result of medical fraud, utilization of unnecessary medical treatments and pharmaceutical companies over charging patients for drugs. The cost of healthcare in the US in 2007 was 2.7 trillion or $7600 per person In 2007, health care spending in the United States reached $2.3 trillion, and was projected to reach $3 trillion in 2011.1 Health care spending is projected to reach $4.2 trillion by 2016. The high cost of prescription drugs has been causing pain and hardships for millions of Americans for years.

Unlike every other advanced country, the United States permits drug companies and pharmacies to charge patients whatever they choose. The United States spends almost $1,000 per person per year on pharmaceuticals. That's around 40 percent more than the next highest spend Prices in the U.S. for brand-name patented drugs are 50 to 60 percent higher than in France and twice as high as in the United Kingdom or Australia. That's because in many countries, government agencies essentially regulate the prices of medicines and set limits to the amount they will reimburse; they may only agree to pay for a drug if they feel that the price is justified by the therapeutic benefits.

Prescription drug prices in the United States have been among the highest in the world. The high cost of prescription drugs became a major topic of discussion in the new millennium, leading up to the U.S. health care reform debate of 2009, and received renewed attention in 2015. High prescription drug prices have been attributed to government-granted monopolies to manufacturers and organizations lacking ability to negotiate prices.

France and Japan demonstrate that it is possible to have cost-containment at the same time as paying physicians using similar tools to those used in the U.S. There are three key things that stand out when you compare these countries to the U.S. They use a common fee schedule so that hospitals, doctors and health services are paid similar rates for most of the patients they see. In the U.S., how much a health care service gets paid depends on the kind of insurance a patient has. This means that health care services can choose patients who have an insurance policy that pays them more generously than other patients who have lower-paying insurers, such as Medicaid.

The most important factor that drives prescription drug prices higher in the United States than anywhere else in the world is the existence of government-protected monopoly rights for drug manufacturers. The FDA has taken a number of significant steps to provide greater access to affordable prescription medications, including unprecedented steps to lower drug costs by helping to speed the development and approval of low-cost generic drugs after legitimate patents have expired on branded drugs. Generic drugs typically cost 50 to 70 percent less than their brand-name counterparts.

On June 18, 2003, the FDA published a final rule to improve access to generic drugs and lower prescription drug costs for millions of Americans. These changes would have saved Americans over $35 billion in drug costs over the 10 years, and would also provide billions in savings for the Medicare and Medicaid programs. Elements of this rule were codified as part of the Medicare law and that, with FDA's technical assistance, the law added additional mechanisms to enhance generic competition in the marketplace.

They are flexible in responding if they think certain costs are exceeding what they budgeted for. In Japan, if spending in a specific area seems to be growing faster than projected, they lower fees for that area. Similarly, in France an organization called CNMATS closely monitors spending across all kinds of services and if they see a particular area is growing faster than they expected (or deem it in the public interest), they can intervene by lowering the price for that service. These countries also supplement lowering fees with other tools.

For example, they monitor how many generic drugs a physician is prescribing and can send someone from the insurance fund to visit physicians' offices to encourage them to use cheaper generic drugs where appropriate. In comparison, U.S. payment rates are much less flexible. They are often statutory and Medicare cannot change the rates without approval by Congress. This makes the system very inflexible for cost containment. There are few methods for controlling rising costs in private insurance in the U.S. In running their business, private health insurers continually face a choice between asking health care providers to contain their costs and passing on higher costs to patients in higher premiums.

Costs could be controlled by: addressing medical fraud, unnecessary treatments and pharmaceutical company profits. Criminal fraud must be factored into the current debates about health care reform, budget deficits, and proposed Medicare/Medicaid cutbacks. As a political entity, how can we make good public policy if we don't know how much of the nation's one trillion dollar health care budget is being lost to fraud?

The amounts are staggering, measured in hundreds of billions of dollars, but nobody knows for sure exactly how much is being lost. Fraud is rampant, largely uncontrolled, and mostly invisible to policymakers. Drug companies are not allowed to promote an "off label" use of its drugs. For instance, if the Food and Drug Administration (FDA) for approval of a certain use of a drug, a pharmaceutical drug company cannot promote another unapproved use. You could be entitled to a large reward if you report off-label drug promotion fraud.

An example would be where the FDA approves drug XYZ to be used to treat epilepsy. Once receiving FDA approval, however, the drug company starts contacting psychiatrists to promote the potential benefits of using drug XYZ for treating depression. The drug company seeks to reap large profits by only asking the FDA to test and approve the drug for a limited area, but then sell millions of pills to doctors to prescribe for other untested uses.

In these troubled times, perhaps no institution has unraveled more quickly and more completely than American medicine. In only a few decades, the medical system has been overrun by organizations seeking to exploit for profit the trust that vulnerable and sick Americans place in their healthcare. Our politicians have proven themselves either unwilling or incapable of reining in the increasingly outrageous costs faced by patients, and market-based solutions only seem to funnel larger and larger sums of our money into the hands of corporations.

A significant segment of the medical industry, it seems, regards fraud and abuse not as a problem, but as a lucrative enterprise worth defending. The managed care environment produces scams involving underutilization, and the withholding of medical care schemes that are harder to uncover and investigate, and much more dangerous to human health.

Health care is a tempting target for thieves. Medicaid pays $415 billion a year; Medicare nearly $600 billion. Total health spending in America is a massive $2.7 trillion, or 17% of GDP. No one knows for sure how much of that is embezzled, but in 2012 Donald Berwick, a former head of the Centres for Medicare and Medicaid Services (CMS), and Andrew Hackbarth of the RAND Corporation, estimated that fraud (and the extra rules and inspections required to fight it) added as much as $98 billion, or roughly 10%, to annual Medicare and Medicaid spending and up to $272 billion across the entire health system.

Doctors, pharmacies, and patients act in league. Scammers over-bill for real services rather than charging for non-existent ones. That makes them harder to spot. Some criminals are switching from cocaine trafficking to prescription-drug fraud because the risk-adjusted rewards are higher: the money is still good, the work safer and the penalties lighter.

Unnecessary health care (overutilization, overuse, or overtreatment) is healthcare provided with a higher volume or cost than is appropriate. Overuse is the predominant factor in its expense, Such factors leave many actors in the system (doctors, patients, pharmaceutical companies, device manufacturers) with inadequate incentive to restrain health care prices or overuse accounting for about a third of healthcare spending in the US ($750 billion out of $2.6 trillion).

Pharmaceutical companies paid $6.6 billion in 2012 to settle claims that they defrauded federal and state government health programs. That's more than double the amount of all settlements in 2011. Drug companies have paid a total of $1.6 billion since 2001 to settle seven suits brought by whistle-blowers that accused them of marketing fraud and overbilling Medicare and Medicaid, according to a report released yesterday by an advocacy group.

The drug industry has now become the biggest defrauder of the federal government, as determined by payments it has made for violations of the False Claims Act (FCA), surpassing the defense industry, which had long been the leader, according to a new Public Citizen study. Desperate to maintain their high margin of profit in the face of a dwindling number of important new drugs, these figures show that the pharmaceutical industry has engaged in such activities as dangerous, illegal promotion for unapproved uses of drugs. Many drug companies say they charge these prices to cover the costs of research and development. But the reality is that many companies are spending more on advertising than they are on these other expenses.

How much should drug companies charge, who should decide and how? And how much is too much? More transparency is desperately needed. It's worth noting that Big Pharma spends more money lobbying American politicians than any other industry.

Health care consumers need to identify these health care fraudsters and report them to attempt to salvage the health care system. People need to remember that he/she could receive a monetary reward for being a whistle blower.

Whistle blowers are people who expose unethical or illegal wrongdoing within companies by reporting it internally to superiors or externally to the media, government authorities, or specialized attorneys. They can be either current or past employees (insiders), or outside individuals who are familiar with the unlawful conduct, and are not required to be U.S. citizens. If you properly report Medicare fraud, you may be entitled to a significant whistleblower reward.

17. Optometry Fraud

Optometry is a health care profession which involves examining the eyes and applicable visual systems for defects or abnormalities as well as the medical diagnosis and management of eye disease. Traditionally, the field of optometry began with the primary focus of correcting refractive error through the use of spectacles.

Modern day optometry, however, has evolved through time so that the educational curriculum additionally includes intensive medical training in the diagnosis and management of ocular disease in countries where the profession is established and regulated. Optometry is a healthcare profession that is autonomous, educated, and regulated (licensed/registered), and optometrists are the primary healthcare practitioners of the eye and visual system who provide comprehensive eye and vision care, which includes refraction and dispensing, detection/diagnosis and management of disease in the eye, and the rehabilitation of conditions of the visual system

One optometrist frequently visited area nursing homes and often claimed to treat more than 100 nursing-home patients in a single day. The complaint alleges that on certain dates, these services would have required more than 20 hours' worth of direct patient care per day, and that the optometrist was not working inside these nursing homes more than 8 hours per day.

The complaint against the optometrist claims that the defendants sought payment for routine monthly eye examinations that were unreasonable and unnecessary given the patients' conditions. Many nursing-home patients received an eye examination from this optometrist every four to five weeks for five years or more. At times, he billed Medicare for certain eye examinations more than any other optometrist in the United States.

Evidence presented at today's guilty plea hearing showed that an optometrist, and an owner of a optometry practice submitted claims to Medicare for payment for eye examinations of nursing-home patients. Instead of billing Medicare for the actual service he was providing at the nursing homes, he claimed that he was conducting the most expensive type of eye examination, which typically lasts 45 minutes.

An example of this health care fraud presented at today's guilty plea hearing involved a July 27, 2009 visit by the optometrist to a nursing home in Georgia, where he billed Medicare for 177 patients whom he claimed to have examined individually for 45 minutes each during that one-day visit. As a result of this type of fraudulent billing, Medicare paid that optometrist for that type of eye exam more than any other doctor in the United States in 2009.

An optometrist must pay $283,499 to settle government allegations that he wrongfully submitted claims to Medicaid for bifocal lenses, trifocal lenses and new patient visits. He was also accused of billing Medicaid, Medicare and TRICARE for medically unnecessary visual field examinations from June 1, 2006, through Dec. 31, 2012. Authorities have filed felony charges against an optometrist who worked in Montana for allegedly submitting false insurance claims. Authorities believe that in numerous instances he billed for eye photography that wasn't necessary. He's also accused of diagnosing some patients with benign neoplasm when they did not, in fact, have the condition.

The optometrist and his business wrongly received more than $1 million from Medicaid and Medicare through the submission of false and inflated bills, federal prosecutors allege in a complaint filed in U.S. District Court in Tulsa.

A lawsuit claims that the federal government lost $846,967 due to an optometrist's submission of hundreds of bills that claimed excessive hours worked. In one instance, the federal government claims, he billed Medicare for 68 hours of work on one day. In all, the lawsuit claims that he billed Medicare in excess of 12 hours per day on 387 occasions, with 124 in excess of 24 hours per day. The billings are "a further indication that the defendant did not provide the required medical services and did not spend the 'face-to-face' time required" to justify the billing under the codes that were submitted, according to the lawsuit.

Although fee-splitting was once universally condemned as unethical, the government-sanctioned "optometric-ophthalmic comanagement," which permits the splitting of the fee for performing cataract surgery. Ophthalmologists retain 80 percent of the government-approved fee, and optometrists receive 20 percent. The result is that whenever the optometrist refers a patient for cataract surgery, the optometrist receives the equivalent of a kickback from the ophthalmologist for postoperative management. The Government has rationalized this arrangement on the grounds that optometrists are qualified to provide postoperative care and merit 20 percent of the surgeon's fee for doing so.

However, the reality is quite different. Optometrists are paid 20 percent of the surgeon's fee for referring a patient to a relatively small group of ophthalmologists willing to participate in the kickback scheme. This represents a generous government-provided stipend to optometrists for making a telephone call and prescribing a pair of glasses. Not all optometrists

A jury could hear the case of a pharmacist and doctor arrested on prescription fraud and drug charges. From his former shop in Kokomo, an optometrist landed him and a pharmacist in jail. The optometrist went to a K-Mart pharmacy and had a prescription filed. However, the optometrist, wasn't authorized to write prescriptions for controlled substances. He prescribed glasses.

There were DEA numbers on the prescriptions that were assigned to other physicians, some assigned to drug stores, The doctor basically stole other doctor's identities, police say, and prescriptions were filled in the name of other patients. But the optometrist always walked into the pharmacy, and the pharmacist always filled the prescriptions. The optometrist had a legitimate prescription for the painkiller OxyContin, police say, which he allegedly traded for another drug with a woman in Grant County. An undercover agent later bought that OxyContin.

"Pretty regular pattern," a prosecutor said. "The undercover officer actually was at the store and witnessed the transaction."

The government also alleges that because of the high number of patients seen by an optometrist on a daily basis, that it was not possible for all of the patients to receive a legitimate eye exam. Therefore, the exams had no medical value. A billing company billed Medicare and Medicaid for all eye examinations provided by an optometrist to nursing-home patients and received payment from those programs.

The manager of an Oklahoma City optometry clinic which closed in October has now been charged with sixteen counts of Medicaid fraud. After an investigation by the agency's Medicaid Fraud Unit, the Oklahoma Attorney General's Office filed charges against the optometrist. Another optometrist is accused of billing the Oklahoma Health Care Authority (OHCA), which oversees state, purchased insurance Sooner Care (Oklahoma Medicaid), for eyeglasses that were never made or delivered to patients. The charges accuse the optometrist of making $359,459 in fraudulent claims since June 2011, billing the OHCA for 3,496 pairs of glasses when only 524 were manufactured and delivered to patients. Prosecutors allege that this optometrist billed for an additional 57 pairs of glasses after the clinic closed.

Another optometrist who managed his father's now-defunct optometry clinic, billed the Oklahoma Health Care Authority $353,830.31 for 2,922 pairs of eye glasses that were never made, records show. This optometrist generated false claims for eye glasses purportedly provided to Medicaid recipients when, in reality, no glasses were manufactured or delivered. This optometrist submitted the fraudulent claims between June 1, 2011, and Nov. 1, 2012, without his father's knowledge.

From January 2007 through January 2012, a Kentucky optometrist provided, or claimed to provide eye examinations and other optometric services to Medicare and Kentucky Medicaid beneficiaries residing in nursing homes in the eastern part of Kentucky. The lawsuit also states that the billing company submitted those claims for payment for his actual or alleged optometric services.

Another complaint alleges that irrespective of condition or diagnosis, the optometrist in question provided eye examinations to most of his nursing-home patients on a monthly basis, a frequency that was unreasonable and unnecessary given the patients' medical conditions. A federal grand jury has charged a Caldwell optometrist with swindling more than $1 million from health care benefit programs. The optometrist allegedly lied and submitted false material to several programs, especially to Medicaid and Medicare. He dishonestly billed the programs, the indictment says, for false diagnoses, including glaucoma, color blindness, tension headaches and treatment of eye injuries.

The indictment further alleges that although he treated only 3.9 percent of Idaho's Medicaid clients from Jan. 1, 2004 to May 8, 2009 he reported diagnosing 99 percent of all acquired color deficiency cases among Idaho Medicaid patients. He also diagnosed 92 percent of all glaucomatous atrophy (optic cupping) cases and 86 percent of all chronic angle closure glaucoma cases. It is also alleged that, in 2008, this optometrist learned about the federal investigation, abruptly stopped submitting claims for glaucoma-related services and began billing for a variety of new diagnoses.

Health care consumers need to identify these health care fraudsters and report them to attempt to salvage the health care system. People need to remember that he/she could receive a monetary reward for being a whistle blower.

Whistle blowers are people who expose unethical or illegal wrongdoing within companies by reporting it internally to superiors or externally to the media, government authorities, or specialized attorneys. They can be either current or past employees (insiders), or outside individuals who are familiar with the unlawful conduct, and are not required to be U.S. citizens. If you properly report Medicare fraud, you may be entitled to a significant whistleblower reward.

18. Chiropractic Fraud

Wikipedia defines chiropractic as a form of alternative medicine mostly concerned with the diagnosis and treatment of mechanical disorders of the musculoskeletal system, especially the spine. Proponents claim that such disorders affect general health via the nervous system.

Daniel David Palmer discovered the power of spinal manipulation by allegedly healing a deaf man by repositioning a vertebra in his spine. Shortly after, he healed someone with heart trouble through the same technique. Convinced he discovered a new medical technique, he opened the Palmer School of Chiropractic in 1897. Palmer claimed that 95% of all diseases were caused by displaced vertebrae, a belief many chiropractors today still hold. To explain this, he invented new terms like "subluxation" (a displacement of the spine). Chiropractors believe bones can get subtly out of line and cause muscle spasms or nerve irritation. This causes the pain. Realigning the bones by manipulations called adjustments supposedly helps relieve it.

Further, most chiropractors claim their adjustments do more than just relieve pain; they allow the body to function better. If nerves aren't being pinched, all messages they transmit, from digestion to muscle relaxation to hormonal activation, can proceed more normally. Chiropractic researchers have documented that fraud, abuse and quackery are more prevalent in chiropractic than in other health care professions. A study of California disciplinary statistics during 1997–2000 reported 4.5 disciplinary actions per 1000 chiropractors per annum, compared to 2.27 for medical doctors, and the incident rate for fraud was nine times greater among chiropractors (1.99 per 1000 chiropractors per annum than among medical doctors.

Chiropractic therapy was established as a profession in 1895. It is now the second-largest primary health-care field in the world. You may be scared of the dangers and side effects of pills and procedures that may lead you to seek out chiropractic therapy. Chiropractic therapy as a profession emphasizes your body's natural health abilities. Many people associate chiropractic therapy with only back and neck pain. However, chiropractic therapy has been shown to be safe for the treatment of headaches, carpal tunnel syndrome, and pain in your arms and legs.

Low back pain may have many causes. In most cases of injury or strain, it takes time for your back to heal. Back pain lasts just as long if you go to a chiropractor, if you go to a physical therapist, or if you seek no treatment at all. Chiropractic manipulation and conventional medical care are about equally effective for relieving acute low back pain. Chiropractic treatment is based upon the concept that restricted movement in the spine may lead to pain and reduced function.

Spinal adjustment is just one form of therapy chiropractors use to treat restricted spinal mobility. During an adjustment, chiropractors use their hands to apply a controlled, sudden force to a joint. Chiropractors may also use massage and stretching to relax muscles that are shortened or in spasm. Many use additional treatments as well, such as ultrasound, electrical muscle stimulation and exercises.

Chiropractic medicine can improve your body function and enhance your body's healing powers. Some chiropractors emphasize a healthy lifestyle, a healthful diet, and stress reduction. They will educate you with respect to your lifestyle at each visit. Many times you doctor will refer you to a chiropractor or physical therapist if you have neck and back pain. In many instances, your doctor will refer you to a chiropractor, who often works together with a physical therapist working at their clinic. Both professions can help you with your chronic pain.

The definition of chiropractic therapy is the correction of problems that exist in your spinal column. This enables your body to function at its peak level without medications, surgical procedures, or steroid injections. In 1999, more than 25 million Americans were treated by chiropractors. Not only do chiropractors take care of back injuries; they also can help you with your neck, hip, leg, ankle, foot, arm, and hand pain. Most back and neck pains are the result of mechanical disorders in your spine.

The problem with chiropractic medicine is that it has been maligned for a long time in the United States. However, it is now widely accepted. In Canada, which is under a national health-care system, chiropractic care is included among treatment methods that are reimbursed by the national system. If you have a back injury caused by a twist or turn, you may want to go to a chiropractor. If you have a back injury and need strengthening exercises, your doctor may refer you to a physical therapist.

Chiropractic medicine focuses attention on the relationship between the structure of your spine and how it affects your nervous system. If your spine is not in alignment due to slouching or poor posture, this can cause some of your nerves to be compressed by your spine. Your chiropractor will adjust your spine to remove any spinal abnormalities to reduce pressure off of the nerves in your arms and legs. When your spine is not aligned correctly, it can cause you to experience tension in your muscles that will in turn affect your nervous system (spinal cord and the nerves emerging from your spinal cord). Compression on your spine and the nerves that come off of your spinal cord can cause you significant health problems and pain. In many instances, an adjustment of your spine can remedy these problems.

Following your initial care, your chiropractor may re-evaluate your progress from time to time. After your spine has been misaligned for any length of time, your body may have a tendency to resume that misalignment again. Therefore, periodic visits with your chiropractor are recommended.

Traction is another method that is frequently used by chiropractors and physical therapists and can be an effective treatment for back pain. Traction involves mechanical forces that separate adjacent body parts away from each other. If you have problems with a disc in your neck or back, traction can separate the bones in your back and increase your blood flow to your injured disc, which can speed up the healing process. If traction worsens of your pain, you should inform your health-care provider so that the traction can be immediately discontinued. Because of the differences in muscle mass between men and women, the amount of traction applied will differ between men and women. If you have a ruptured disc in your neck or back, traction can help heal this painful entity.

Chiropractors treat other entities besides back pain. For example, if you have a carpal tunnel syndrome, chiropractic manipulation can sometimes correct this condition. On occasion, you may not need surgery after chiropractic treatment. Given that no two people are alike, if you are taking any medications and begin to take nutritional supplements you should be aware that potential drug-nutrient interactions may occur and are encouraged to consult a health-care professional before using any natural product. Combining certain prescription drugs and dietary supplements can lead to undesirable effects such as: diminished prescription-drug effectiveness, reduced supplement effectiveness and impaired drug and/or supplement absorption.

Chiropractic and nutritional treatment contribute to the amelioration and perhaps reversal of osteoarthritis (OA). It is further proposed that the chiropractic manipulative thrust, is, in effect, treating dysfunctional bio-mechanics of joints, affecting positive cartilaginous change. The pathophysiology and multi-factorial causes of OA are reviewed. New interpretations of the literature surrounding OA are discussed, which offer arguments for OA's treatment and reversal through chiropractic manipulation and nutritional support.

Some chiropractors recommend DRX 9000 machine treatments. The DRX 9000 is a traction table billed by those who treat back pain (mainly chiropractors and in an area of a group of DO's) as a spinal "decompression" unit. I initially became suspicious and concerned about the device when I had several back pain patients who were previously treated at the DO's facility. They all said that their treatment consisted of daily treatments for six weeks of spinal decompression in the DRX 9000, water massage and blowing up a balloon. Regardless if patients had simple mechanical low back pain, a herniated disc, spinal stenosis, etc., everyone received the same treatment. The worst part is, in many cases, their insurance companies did not pay for this plan of care.

A Wichita, Kansas, a chiropractor pleaded guilty to one count of health care fraud, two counts of aggravated identity theft and one count of tax evasion. In his plea, he admitted that from March 2011 to October 2013, he executed a health care fraud scheme through his businesses. He submitted false claims to Medicare, Blue Cross/Blue Shield of Kansas and Coventry Health Care of Kansas, Inc., and the Federal Employees Health Benefits Program.

Chiropractors have a limited scope of practice. They are not allowed to perform injections, dispense drugs or supervise ARNPs and physicians. A chiropractor developed what he called an "integrated practice," hiring physicians, advanced registered nurse practitioners and physical therapists and ostensibly having them perform procedures he was not qualified to perform. He misrepresented to the Kansas Board of Healing Arts that medical doctors had an ownership in his clinic. He used the names of physicians he employed to submit false claims for services. This chiropractor fraudulently billed for nerve conduction tests, nerve block injections, subcutaneous infiltrate proceedings, fine needle aspirations and ultrasound procedures.

A chiropractic scheme perpetuated involved paying individuals to stage accidents, and then report to the clinics with a list of symptoms that they were coached to provide. Various accusations were made in court documents, including: having patients sign bills for numerous dates of service when treatment was not rendered, up coding exams and billing for more services than provided. The clinic submitted almost $40,000 in fraudulent insurance claims to six separate insurance companies. An owner of a local collision repair shop was paid to provide patients (motor vehicle accidents) for a referral fee.

More than 36,000 chiropractors were paid nearly $500 million by the federal government in 2012, making chiropractors one of the largest groups of Medicare providers. And one chiropractor in Brooklyn topped the list, receiving more than $1 million that year alone. Overall, chiropractors provided 21 million taxpayer-funded treatments for 2.5 million beneficiaries; the Medicare data show. But just 600 chiropractors accounted for more than 10% of the Medicare payments.

Many patients report being told that because they have pain, an x-ray is warranted. While pain is one of the criteria that can constitute the need for an x-ray, it is not, in and of itself, enough. An x-ray should only be taken if your history leads the physician to believe that you may have serious spinal pathology, or if the patient has already undergone 4-6 weeks of conservative care without satisfactory improvement.

Another way that x-rays can be detrimental has to do with how they are used rather than any exposure to radiation. Many physicians like to sit down and show each patient their study, including the x-ray images. And while this seems like a commendable thing for a physician to do, there are studies indicate that showing a patient their x-rays can decrease their rate of progress.

Some chiropractic and pain physicians will take this one step further. They will show a patient all the areas of degeneration and tell them that the degeneration is causing the pain. However, leading studies to refute this idea and show that mild to moderate degeneration does not cause pain. Even though this information has been available for some time, many physicians continue to blame low back pain on degeneration when the fact is that there are many people out there with no back pain that have degeneration. In addition, as you age, you are more likely to have degeneration; therefore, the majority of the time, the x-ray ends up illustrating what was already known and does not change the treatment.

Over the past few years non-surgical spinal decompression devices have become the latest trend within the Chiropractic field. Insurance companies do not cover this procedure in many instances. Therefore, patients need to pay for this treatment out of pocket with no guarantees. Many doctors only bill the insurance company if the patient has insurance and no ability to pay. This is accomplished by using fraudulent codes in order to obtain payment. Non-surgical spinal decompression devices can very well cause further injuries.

Chiropractic often involves many expensive but quick treatments and marketing and sales tactics that many people consider to be aggressive and distasteful, if not downright unethical, especially pre-paid treatment packages, and the emphasis of many other services and products. A 2016 federal US audit concluded that more than 80% Medicare payments to chiropractors were for medically unnecessary procedures and 100% of treatments were unnecessary after the first thirty.

Two chiropractors were indicted by a federal grand jury in Georgia on charges of health care fraud. .S. Attorney for the Northern District of Georgia, said during that time, the chiropractors billed Blue Cross/Blue Shield of Georgia for approximately $633,990 based on vertebral axial decompression, a mechanical procedure performed on patients. The insurance company considered the procedure to be not medically necessary. The chiropractors instructed employees at the Back Pain Institute of Columbus to alter the patient files to hide the use of VAX-D from Blue Cross, and to bill the insurer for other medically covered procedures.

A Camden County chiropractor is facing up to five years in prison after admitting that he defrauded insurance companies of more than $6,400 reimbursed for treatments he never provided to patients, authorities said. The investigation also implicated Camden police officers accused of illegally obtaining accident reports and delivering them to American Spinal Care for use to solicit business, authorities said.

The New Jersey Manufacturers Insurance Co. said that it has filed suit to try to recoup hundreds of thousands of dollars paid in allegedly bogus medical claims. The civil suit, filed last week in Superior Court in Trenton, names 55 claimants as defendants for allegedly faking injuries and 11 health care companies and three doctors as "defendants in interest" because they collected money on the claims. The insurer alleges that claimants, primarily from the Irvington area, had pretended to be accident victims between November 2000 and August 2004 and received diagnostic tests and medical treatment. The accidents "either never occurred or were staged," The claims indicated little or no damage to the vehicles, but multiple passengers complained of injuries requiring medical treatment. Many of the defendants sought care at the same chiropractic centers and were represented by the same lawyers, the insurer said in the news release.

A Deputy District Attorney said a chiropractor provided weekly chiropractic treatments for her husband and two children for several years, then turned in claim forms that said the services were provided by another employee. The claimant's insurance policy does not cover treatments done by a family member.

A chiropractor in Tampa, Florida would pay patients up to $1,000 each to come to his clinic for "treatment." He would then bill each individual's insurance company for nonexistent treatments." He was subsequently charged with three counts of patient brokering. Chiropractic therapy can be beneficial for the management of some chronic pain conditions. However, a potential patient should seek the services of a reputable and honest chiropractor before consenting to treatment.

Health care consumers need to identify these health care fraudsters and report them to attempt to salvage the health care system. People need to remember that he/she could receive a monetary reward for being a whistle blower.

Whistle blowers are people who expose unethical or illegal wrongdoing within companies by reporting it internally to superiors or externally to the media, government authorities, or specialized attorneys. They can be either current or past employees (insiders), or outside individuals who are familiar with the unlawful conduct, and are not required to be U.S. citizens. If you properly report Medicare fraud, you may be entitled to a significant whistleblower reward.

19. Medical Research Fraud

Biomedical research (or experimental medicine) is in general simply known as medical research. It is the basic research, applied research, or translational research conducted to aid and supports the development body of knowledge in the field of medicine. Fraud and misconduct in clinical research is widespread. Only 2% of scientists admit to fabricating or falsifying data. But 14% said that they had personal evidence of such behavior in their colleagues, suggesting that it is underreported

The US Food and Drug Administration (FDA) is responsible for protecting public health by assuring the safety and efficacy of drugs, biological products, medical devices, food, and more. Much has been written about research fraud and there have been many high-profile cases. But of great concern to us are the direct victims of the fraud: patients given inappropriate treatment or denied full safety assessment while taking an experimental drug. Then there are the invisible victims, patients of a doctor removed from practice having been found guilty of research fraud. We'd like to share the stories of some of these victims.

Many protocols require patients to be treatment-naïve or uncontrolled on present medication. When patients were interviewed in a depression study, patient notes were altered to make it appear that the patient fitted the inclusion criteria. The records showed that a husband and wife participated in the same study. Both agreed that they had been asked to take part in the study, both discussed participation, and both had signed consent forms.

The husband was asked, what was his history of depression? "I've never been depressed in my life!" he responded. He had had a miserable 12 weeks with every known side effect. His wife, however, complained that she had received no benefit whatsoever from being in the study. He had received the active medication, and she had received a placebo. She was denied medication, and he was treated for a condition he did not have. Furthermore, his medical notes now show that he suffered from depression, which may influence future choices of treatment, employment, and insurance.

Another researcher falsified the results of several vaccine experiments supported by grants from the US National Institutes of

Health (NIH). In some cases, this researcher spiked rabbit blood samples with human HIV antibodies so that the vaccine appeared to have caused the animals to develop immunity to the virus.

Different forms of fraud (e.g., fabrication and falsification of data, deceptive reporting of results, suppression of data, and deceptive design or analysis) were observed in fairly similar numbers. Sometimes, the impact on patients can be financial as well as a loss of trust.

New drug development revolves around the need to show efficacy, safety, and quality. Unless all three are measured accurately, any conclusions will be false. A clinical research associate revealed that her research unit had many studies with insufficient research staff, and she couldn't do all the tests laid down in the various protocols on all the patients. So she made up some of the data. This was a drug just starting its course through Phase III, with much still unknown about its safety and efficacy.

Drug companies bribe researchers and doctors as a routine matter. Medical journals routinely publish false, fraudulent studies. FDA panel members regularly rely on falsified research in making their drug approval decisions, and the mainstream media regularly quotes falsified research in reporting the news.

Pfizer paid $73,512 for a study of the use of Celebrex in post-operative pain, but the doctor doing the study made up his results, according to federal prosecutors. It is a system operated by criminals who fabricate whatever "scientific evidence" they need in order to get published in medical journals and win FDA approval for drugs that they fully realize are killing people. Dr. Scott Reuben, a former member of Pfizer's speakers' bureau, has agreed to plead guilty to faking dozens of research studies that were published in medical journals.

Now being reported across the mainstream media is the fact that Dr. Reuben accepted a $75,000 grant from Pfizer to study Celebrex in 2005. His research, which was published in a medical journal, has since been quoted by hundreds of other doctors and researchers as "proof" that Celebrex helped reduce pain during post-surgical recovery. There's only one problem with all this: No patients were ever enrolled in the study!

Another researcher was paid by leading drug companies such as Novartis and Sanofi to conduct trials of antipsychotic drugs on patients with schizophrenia and Alzheimer's. According to the General Medical Council (GMC), he recruited people in unsolicited telephone calls without contacting vulnerable patients' psychiatric nurses; he failed to obtain proper approval from ethical committees to conduct a number of major studies; he used the same patients as subjects for a number of different studies thereby invalidating the studies for which he had been paid hundreds of thousands of dollars. The GMC panel found this researcher to be responsible for conducting research without appropriate human subjects' approvals; improperly presenting himself as having a PhD; and selling drugs he got for free from drug companies for his research to hospitals.

Recently, Merck has been in the firing line for allegedly fraudulently representing the mumps component of its MMR vaccine. It has been alleged that Merck had been fraudulently informing the public that the MMR II, used to replace the MMR vaccine Pluserix, is an effective vaccine when this is not true because the studies proving the vaccine's effectiveness is said to be falsified.

GlaxoSmithKline came under scrutiny as well. The drug giant plead guilty to promoting two drugs for unapproved uses and failing to report safety data about a diabetes drug to the Food and Drug Administration (FDA). The settlement will cover criminal fines as well as civil settlements with the federal and state governments. The case concerns the drugs Paxil, Wellbutrin and Avandia.

According to news reports, Celebrex is no better at protecting the stomach from serious complications than other drugs. Pfizer and its partner, Pharmacia, were able to misrepresent Celebrex as a safer alternative because they only released the results of half of a yearlong study.

Abbott Laboratories pleaded guilty and agreed to pay $1.5 billion for unlawfully promoting the prescription-drug Depakote for uses not approved safe and effective by the Food and Drug Administration (FDA). The FDA originally approved the drug for epileptic seizures, bipolar mania and the prevention of migraines. The press release clearly states that this drug was never approved for controlling behavioral disturbances in dementia patients. This was because the drug was found to be dangerous in elderly patients causing some of them to suffer from dehydration and anorexia after using this drug.

Actos, which is manufactured by Takeda Pharmaceuticals, has been used by thousands of patients in the U.S. to help treat diabetes. However, after further studies revealed that the drug was linked to increasing one's risk of developing bladder cancer.

Though the reported fraud does not invalidate other studies on the health benefits of resveratrol, it nevertheless, gives an unwarranted black eye to a promising compound which other studies have indicated is anti-inflammatory, cardio-protective, prevents cancer, increases energy, lowers blood sugar and extends life.

Major studies within cancer research have been proven to be false, which suggests that the mainstream treatments we use are based on fraudulent findings and false science. Recent news has shown that the majority of studies geared towards cancer research are inaccurate and likely fraudulent by nature. Findings published in the journal Nature show that 88% of major studies on cancer that have been published in reputable journals over the years cannot be reproduced to show their accuracy. This means that the research findings published are not based on accurate results.

The author of the review and former head of cancer research at Amgen C. Glenn Begley was unable to replicate the results of 47 of the 53 studies he examined. This suggests that researchers may be fabricating their findings simply to create the illusion of positive findings instead of publishing their actual results. This ensures the continuation of their steady stream of funding and grants. Begley stated: "These are the studies the pharmaceutical industry relies on to identify new targets for drug development, but if you're going to place a $1 million or $2 million or $5 million bet on an observation, you need to be sure it's true. As we tried to reproduce these papers we became convinced you can't take anything at face value."

The University of Michigan's Comprehensive Cancer Center published an analysis in 2009, which revealed popular cancer studies to be false. Unsurprisingly the primary cause of fabricated results was determined to be conflicts of interest that created results that work out best for drug companies rather than for the people.

Health care consumers need to identify these health care fraudsters and report them to attempt to salvage the health care system. People need to remember that he/she could receive a monetary reward for being a whistle blower.

Whistle blowers are people who expose unethical or illegal wrongdoing within companies by reporting it internally to superiors or externally to the media, government authorities, or specialized attorneys. They can be either current or past employees (insiders), or outside individuals who are familiar with the unlawful conduct, and are not required to be U.S. citizens. If you properly report Medicare fraud, you may be entitled to a significant whistleblower reward.

20. Dentistry Fraud

Dentistry is a branch of medicine that is involved in the study, diagnosis, prevention, and treatment of diseases, disorders and conditions of the oral cavity, commonly in the dentition but also the oral mucosa, and of adjacent and related structures and tissues, particularly in the maxillofacial (jaw and facial) area. It's only a small percentage of providers or consumers who commit healthcare fraud, but that small percentage can have a big impact. The U.S. spends more than $2 trillion on healthcare annually. At least 3 percent of that spending or $68 billion is lost to fraud each year.

Most dentists are honest, ethical professionals who provide their patients competent and caring treatment. A small but disturbing number of dentists, however, are dishonest. They exploit their position of authority to bilk trusting patients with useless and often painful treatment, and shady billing practices.

Dishonest dentists perform useless surgery on perfectly healthy patients to increase their own insurance billings. The fraudulent dentists remove healthy teeth, do root canals that aren't needed, and drill for cavities that don't exist. Sometimes children's teeth are even drilled without a painkiller. Often the surgery is inferior. Shoddy crowns or fillings fall out. Patients have found surgical debris embedded in their gums. Patients also become painfully infected and disfigured, and need more surgery to correct the treatments.

Dishonest dentists do minor procedures such as routine tooth cleanings, but bill your insurance plan for costlier treatments such as phantom root canals or cavity fillings. Fraudulent dentists bill insurers for treatments they never performed. They send the insurer forged bills for fake treatment, medicine and supplies they never used. They may bill the policies of current patients, or invent "patients" they've never even met.

Sometimes dentists illegally treat patients despite losing their licenses for previous infractions. Some dentists also have hygienists; assistants or other staff perform treatments even though they aren't licensed or qualified. The dentists then bill insurers as if the dentists performed the treatment themselves.

Examples of fraudulent dental practices include: Dental offices that routinely fail to charge or collect your full coinsurance or copayment amount or deductible. This amounts to overbilling the insurance company for the services rendered. Dentists that perform unnecessary treatment (e.g. x-rays, fillings and crowns) that aren't needed. Patients or dental offices that conceal another patient insurance coverage, Incorrect information placed on your notice of payment, Individuals who use someone else's identification number, Patients who persuade the dental office to falsify the date of treatment and dental offices that submit a claim for a covered service, when actually a non-covered service was performed.

The most frequent dental scams are inflating claims, delivering worthless treatment that patients don't need and billing insurers for phantom treatment that the dentist never delivered. Some dentists have chosen to inflate their prices, and prey on the unwary by using tactics such as the "old bait and switch" scam. Patients come to their offices for advertised services for an advertised dollar amount and are instead are talked into much higher services when they are told they have a need for braces, extractions, deep cleaning, gum treatment, mouthwashes, expensive night guards, fillings, root canals, crowns, dental posts and retainers.

A dentist billed for procedures where the doctor allegedly used IV sedation, but he would apparently bill Medicaid for the medication under a different provider ID in the amount of up to $2,049 for the service and sent the money directly to his home. He would refer to coding a procedure as having a more extensive degree of difficulty than actually performed. For example: A patient receives a standard prophylaxis examination, but the insurance carrier was billed for periodontal scaling and root planning.

Patient co-payments are considered to be an essential element in the cost structure of the contract between an insurance carrier and whoever is purchasing the coverage. Waiving co-payments are thought to encourage more usage of the coverage than would normally occur,

The correct date a procedure is performed is important as related to patient eligibility requirements and waiting periods. It is fraudulent to send in a claim for a treatment using a date other than the actual date of service.

A problem was brought to light in March 2008 experiencing treatment in a clinic in Maryland. A 4-year-old boy was restrained in a "papoose board "writhing and screaming in pain while undergoing treatment that he did not need. It also shows how the clinic staff members were preoccupied with making money.

ABC-TV's "20/20" aired additional findings in March 2009. These graphic reports show how children were unnecessarily restrained, inadequately anesthetized, and subjected to unnecessary procedures, including multiple tooth removal and tooth capping, that left them psychologically traumatized as well as physically and cosmetically damaged.

Two children shown in the "20/20" report had 16 pulpectomies (root canals) performed at one sitting. The staff was seen choking children to the point of unconsciousness rather than using appropriate anesthetic prior to doing tooth extractions. The dentist was seen performing non-medically necessary dental procedures without anesthetics and was fraudulently billing Medicaid for these procedures using fear and threats to scare and thereby silence his victims, including threats not limited to saying things like 'Your mom will die' if you tell her what happened."

Charges exceeding the amount the dentist submitted to the insurance company is a violation of the contract between an insurance company and the dental office. Most insurance companies expect the patient to pay a portion of the fee (co pay). Just because a dentist accepts a certain insurance plan does not necessarily mean they are contracted with that insurance company. If a dentist accepts an insurance plan, but is not contracted with them, then the dentist will submit their usual and customary fee (which can be higher than a contracted fee) to the insurance company. The insurance then pays the dentist whatever is dictated by the patent's plan and the patient is responsible to pay the difference.

Diagnoses of cavities when none exist may happen as well (E.g. "you have seven cavities"). This is particularly problematic because once a hole has been drilled, the evidence is gone. Also some dentists have different opinions of what needs a filling. Some dentists prefer to watch very small cavities (in hopes that they don't spread) and some dentists like to restore very small cavities.

Charging for multiple cleanings or only cleaning half of a patient's mouth. Sometimes the dentist or hygienist needs more than one hour to remove all the tartar from your teeth. Most insurance companies only cover 1 cleaning every six months, and the patient has to pay out of pocket for the second cleaning. This is very frustrating to the patient if it is not explained; however, it does not constitute fraud. Not releasing records or x-rays to the patient is not fraudulent. It is customary for dental offices to charge a nominal fee (usually about $30) for the duplication of x-rays. Dentists are required to release these records upon written request of the patient; however, they are not required to do so for free.

According to prosecutors, a dentist stole more than $200,000 by submitting hundreds of reimbursement claims to the Medicaid program that falsely stated he had provided such dental services as fillings and cleanings to Medicaid recipients when, in fact, the procedures were unlawfully performed by three employees, including the office manager who were not licensed to practice dentistry.

Sometimes patients want restorations that are considered cosmetic, and insurance companies will not authorize such procedures. Dentists submit fraudulent narratives stating that "leaking" or "broken margins" are present. There is also the ever popular "cracked tooth syndrome" and "failing" restorations and crowns, which can be used to scam the insurance companies.

Health care consumers need to identify these health care fraudsters and report them to attempt to salvage the health care system. People need to remember that he/she could receive a monetary reward for being a whistle blower.

Whistle blowers are people who expose unethical or illegal wrongdoing within companies by reporting it internally to superiors or externally to the media, government authorities, or specialized attorneys. They can be either current or past employees (insiders), or outside individuals who are familiar with the unlawful conduct, and are not required to be U.S. citizens. If you properly report Medicare fraud, you may be entitled to a significant whistleblower reward.

21. Podiatry Fraud

A podiatrist is a doctor of podiatric medicine (DPM), also known as a podiatric physician or surgeon. Podiatrists diagnose and treat conditions of the foot, ankle, and related structures of the leg. The older title of chiropodist may be used by some clinicians. Doctors of podiatric medicine receive medical education and training four years of graduate education at one of nine podiatric medical colleges and up to four years of hospital-based residency training. All podiatric physicians and surgeons receive a DPM degree.

A podiatrist has been indicted for allegedly defrauding Medicare by submitting more than $400,000 in false claims, some for treating patients who don't even have feet. A federal grand jury issued the indictment last week accusing a licensed podiatrist since 1986, of Medicare fraud and 21 counts of making false statements relating to health care matters.

This podiatrist, who saw patients at his Augusta office and at nursing homes in east Georgia and nearby areas in South Carolina, allegedly schemed to defraud Medicare from January 1997 through June 2002, according to the indictment. Documents accused the podiatrist of submitting false claims for treatment of patients who had died and patients, whose feet had been amputated, including one who had been an amputee for nine years. He also is accused of submitting bills for trimming patients' toenails, which is a service not covered by Medicare.

In another case, a foot doctor is among 301 people federally charged Wednesday in the largest Medicare fraud sweep in history. This podiatrist was among 61 doctors charged for allegedly participating in health care fraud schemes totaling some $900 million in false billings. Another 240 nurses and licensed medical professionals also are facing charges. The nationwide sweep is the largest in history by both the total number of defendants charged and loss amount, federal officials said.

He is charged for allegedly participating in a $5 million scheme to defraud Medicare, Medicaid and four private victim insurance companies through his practice in Haverford. According to charging documents, he submitted fraudulent claims for podiatric procedures that were not provided and podiatric procedures that were not performed, including injections, debridement and nail avulsions. He also allegedly submitted fraudulent claims for unnecessary procedures and services that were not reimbursable by Medicare or the other insurance carriers.

The Sixth Circuit on Monday upheld a district court's sentencing of a doctor convicted of participating in a multimillion-dollar false prescription and billing scheme, finding that evidence submitted against her was warranted and that her sentence was just. A three-judge appellate panel found that this individual, a Michigan podiatrist, received a fair trial despite her argument that evidence related to her prescribing of the opiate painkiller hydrocodone would prejudice the jury against her.

The panel also ruled that a pharmacist's testimony about her rate of prescribing the drugs was fairly submitted, and that she couldn't demonstrate how her five-year sentence was unreasonable given the facts of the case. "We discern no abuse of discretion in the evidentiary rulings and conclude that any error in calculating her guidelines range proved harmless," the unsigned opinion said.

Another podiatrist was convicted for her part in a health care fraud conspiracy orchestrated by another individual who is the owner of multiple pharmacies and other health care companies in and around Detroit. The scheme for which 26 individuals were indicted in 2011 involved bribing various physicians and managers of health care companies to write prescriptions for medications with high profit margins that could be billed to Medicare, Medicaid or other insurers.

This podiatrist would then charge insurers for the for the drugs, often shorting patients on medications, including hydrocodone, oxycodone, alprazolam and codeine cough syrup and selling the remainder on the street, according to the opinion. This podiatrist furthermore, proceeded to a jury trial on charges she accepted over $75,000 from another individual to participate in this scheme, and she was ultimately convicted of health care fraud, conspiracy to distribute controlled substances and conspiracy to pay and receive health care kickbacks. She was sentenced to five years in prison and a $4.5 million fine.

On appeal, the podiatrist argued that evidence submitted at trial unfairly biased the jury against her, citing statistics comparing her prescriptions of controlled substances to those of other podiatrists in Michigan and testimony from a pharmacist claiming her prescription rate raised "red flags." However, the panel ruled that the district court did not mistakenly allow the evidence and testimony. The statistics were true and essential to describing her role in the scheme, it said, and the pharmacist was well-positioned to make the statements he did.

In another case a licensed podiatrist, and the office manager, has been arraigned on federal charges of illegal distribution of opioid painkillers and other drugs at clinic locations purporting to provide podiatric care in Georgia. "This podiatrist was trusted to provide appropriate medical care to her patients," said an U. S. Attorney. "Instead, with the assistance of this individual allegedly prescribed addictive opioids without any legitimate medical need. Addiction to powerful prescription opioids unfortunately continues to take a daily toll on many members of our community."

The Special Agent in Charge of the DEA Atlanta Field Division commented upon the case, "It is sad commentary when persons in the medical community abuse their positions of trust to hide behind the veil of legitimacy to commit criminal acts. The reckless distribution of pharmaceuticals results in addiction and death."

According to a U.S. Attorney, the indictment, and other information presented in court stated: that a person in question is a licensed podiatrist, which means she is permitted to evaluate and treat the foot and leg. A nearly three-year federal investigation began after the Georgia Drug & Narcotics Agency (GDNA) visited this doctor in November 2013, and February 2014, to discuss high volume, high dosage prescriptions she had written for opioids. The indictment alleges that despite GDNA's warnings, this doctor, with the assistance of the office managers, continued to prescribe large volumes of controlled substances without a legitimate medical need and outside the scope of a podiatric practice.

For example, during a nine-month period between December 2014 through August 2015, this doctor allegedly prescribed over 116,500 oxycodone 30mg pills, 41,800 hydromorphone 8mg pills, and 400 fentanyl patches. In April 2016, agents with the DEA and HHS executed a federal search warrant at this doctor's office. At that time, the doctor voluntarily surrendered her DEA registration that permitted her to prescribe controlled substances.

The doctor and office manager were both charged with conspiring to distribute controlled substances outside the usual course of professional medical practice and for no legitimate medical purpose from November 2013 to December 2015. The drugs allegedly supplied include oxycodone, hydromorphone, fentanyl, hydrocodone, phentermine, alprazolam, and promethazine with codeine.

This doctor is also charged with two counts of maintaining a podiatry clinic first in Lithonia and later in Sandy Springs for the purpose of illegally distributing drugs. Finally, this podiatrist is charged with fifty-seven individual counts of illegal drug distribution for specific prescriptions written to three separate customers. The office manager is charged with aiding and abetting the doctor for eight of those prescriptions.

Members of the public are reminded that the indictment only contains charges. The defendants are presumed innocent of the charges, and it will be the government's burden to prove the defendants' guilt beyond a reasonable doubt at trial.

In 2007, another podiatrist established a foot and ankle Institute .This practice eventually ran into financial difficulties. This practice hired a podiatrist to work principally in Missouri, though he also provided care in other states. Nine months later, this doctor was indicted on three counts of claiming to treat patients in 2007 and 2008 when he was, in fact, vacationing in Las Vegas and Hawaii. He also provided nursing-home patients care in podiatry, audiology, diagnostics and wound treatment.

According to another indictment, another podiatrist owned podiatry offices located in Michigan, respectively. The indictment alleges that between January 2010 through 2016, this podiatrist falsely conveyed to his podiatry patients that they needed weekly or bi-weekly shots and minor surgeries to prevent hammertoe, which were allegedly medically unnecessary. As a result, these patients returned to his practice on a regular basis every month for shots and minor surgeries. Additionally, this podiatrist allegedly billed Medicare for other podiatry services, such as Unna Boots, which were never given to any of the patients.

Health care consumers need to identify these health care fraudsters and report them to attempt to salvage the health care system. People need to remember that he/she could receive a monetary reward for being a whistle blower.

Whistle blowers are people who expose unethical or illegal wrongdoing within companies by reporting it internally to superiors or externally to the media, government authorities, or specialized attorneys. They can be either current or past employees (insiders), or outside individuals who are familiar with the unlawful conduct, and are not required to be U.S. citizens. If you properly report Medicare fraud, you may be entitled to a significant whistleblower reward.

22. Nurse Fraud

A nurse is a person trained to provide medical care for the sick or disabled, especially one who is licensed and works in a hospital or physician's office. A nurse is a person who is trained to give care (help) to people who are sick or injured. Nurses work with doctors and other health-care workers to make patients well (not sick) and to keep them fit and healthy. Nurses also help with end-of-life needs and assist other family members with grieving.

Nursing is a profession, like a doctor, but training for a nurse is different in how long a person must train and what kind of training they need. In some places, nurses may train for three to five years or more before they get a license as a nurse. Nurses work in many places. Nurses work in hospitals, in doctor's offices, and in the community, and they even visit people at home if they cannot get out.

A Registered Nurse (RN) is a nurse who has graduated from a nursing program and met the requirements outlined by a country, state, province or similar licensing body in order to obtain a nursing license. An RN's scope of practice is determined by legislation, and is regulated by a professional body or council.

Nurses have become heavily involved in a series of health-care-related fraud news in recent years. One of the most controversial reports of fraud from the Department of Justice was in 2011, which involved eight nurses who billed Medicare $18.7 million for services never provided. A former nurse at the hospital has been arrested and charged with numerous crimes related to her alleged use of fraud and forgery to obtain prescription drugs that were intended for patients at the facility.

Patients under the care of a nurse are vulnerable by virtue of illness or injury, and the dependent nature of the nurse-patient relationship. Persons who are especially vulnerable include the elderly, children, the mentally ill, sedated and anesthetized patients, those whose mental or cognitive ability is compromised and patients who are disabled or immobilized.

Patients frequently bring valuables (medications, money, and jewelry, items of sentimental value, checkbook, or credit cards) with them to a health care facility. Nurses frequently provide care in private homes and home-like settings where all of the patient's property and valuables are accessible to the nurse. Nurses frequently provide care in settings without direct supervision.

Theft from a patient raises serious concerns, whether the nurse can be trusted to respect a patient's property/possessions in the future. Theft or deception that occurs outside of the workplace, including conviction or a judicial order involving criminal behavior, may raise concerns as to whether the same misconduct will be repeated in the workplace and, therefore, place patients at risk for theft and deception.

Theft from a patient or engaging in fraudulent or deceitful behavior or conduct with or involving a patient is never acceptable. Theft of patient money, property, medicine, valuables, or items of sentimental value is ground for suspension or revocation of licensure .Massachusetts regulators revoked or suspended the professional licenses of 13 nurses after discovering recently that the health care workers lied about having nursing degrees or being licensed in other states, health department documents show.

A registered nurse who fabricated nursing visit forms in connection with a $24 million home health care fraud conspiracy in Detroit pleaded guilty today for her role in the scheme. She and others conspired to defraud Medicare through home health care companies operating within the Detroit area.

According to court documents, the nurse fabricated nursing visit notes and other documents to give Medicare the impression that she had provided home health care services, when, in fact, home health care was not needed and/or was not being provided. She also admitted that while at these companies, she signed nursing visit notes for home visits made by other unlicensed individuals to give Medicare the false impression that she had provided home health care. Court documents reveal that this nurse understood that the documents she created would be used by these companies to submit claims to Medicare for home-health services that were not medically necessary and/or not provided.

Another individual who operates two nursing agencies was arrested and charged with health care fraud in a criminal complaint. The complaint alleges a scheme to defraud Medicare by billing for unnecessary nursing services that were provided to patients who were not confined to the home and who were obtained via illegal payments for patient referrals. For over three years, beginning in 2011, a total of approximately $5 million was paid to the two agencies by Medicare for services rendered to patients deemed to be homebound.

Seven California residents have pled guilty to forgery charges for using fake transcripts to become licensed registered nurses, following a multiagency probe by the California Department of Consumer Affairs' Division of Investigation (DOI), U.S. Immigration and Customs Enforcement's (ICE) Homeland Security Investigations (HSI) and the Internal Revenue Service (IRS).

According to information presented in court, a registered nurse, owned and operated Mt. Zion Home Health Agency in Denton, Texas. From April 2008 to October 2013, this individual carried out a scheme to defraud Medicare through the submission of false and fraudulent claims for skilled nursing services, which were not provided and, which were not authorized by the patients' physicians.

At times, the nurse submitted claims for services which she allegedly provided when she was out of state. At other times, she submitted claims for services which she allegedly provided to patients who testified that they did not know her and had never heard of her company. She was indicted by a federal grand jury on June 11, 2015.

A registered nurse who bilked an insurance company out of more than $300,000 in workers' compensation benefits was sentenced Tuesday to three years in custody followed by three years of mandatory supervision. She was convicted of a dozen felony counts, including perjury and insurance fraud. She initially told her doctors in January 2007 that she injured her back while waking up from a nightmare.

She initially filed for state disability benefits, but after learning that the most she could receive was $4,515 because she'd only been employed in California for a few months, she filed for workers' compensation benefits. The nurse worked her illegal scam for seven years, defrauding the insurance company and repeatedly lying under oath at her deposition, in her workers' compensation case and to her doctors..

Under workers' compensation benefits, all the defendant's medical expenses were covered, and she received more than $88,000 for the two years she claimed she could not work after her injury. In May 2010, after all conservative care was exhausted, she had back surgery.

A former nurse was arrested after being indicted on a single charge of TennCare Fraud. Investigators with the Tennessee Bureau of Investigation are accusing a nurse with fraud after they reportedly found that she falsified documents and client signatures. According to a news release, investigators with the TBI claim that she falsified timesheets, nursing notes, client signatures and did not work shifts she had reported to her employer.

A nurse pleaded guilty in Bronx Criminal Court Friday to swiping medicinal cocaine from the emergency room at Jacobi Medical Center. This nurse had her license suspended after admitting to stealing the cocaine to feed her personal habit. She got the drugs from a secure medical-storage system by entering the name of a recently discharged patient without the doctor's permission and withdrawing a 4-milliliter vial, according to court papers. She admitted to stealing other drugs, including Oxycodone and Dilaudid on three other occasions.

Another individual, a 77-year-old female and former advanced practice registered nurse (APRN), was arrested by Inspectors from the Medicaid Fraud Control Unit (MCFU) in the Office of the Chief State's Attorney, and charged with one count each of health insurance fraud and making a false prescription.

Over a four-year period beginning in 2010, she wrote more prescriptions than any other health care provider for Vivitrol, an injectable medication used to treat opiate and alcohol addiction and for which the state paid $1,100 or more for each prescription, according to the arrest warrant affidavit.

An investigation by the Drug Control Division in the Department of Consumer Protection found that she wrote nearly 10 times the number of prescriptions as the next highest provider in her state, which was a three-person combined practice. She prescribed Vivitrol on a monthly basis to Medicaid recipients who were either no longer her patients or whom she had never treated.

Over the four-year period under review, the state Department of Social Services paid nearly $2.3 million for the prescriptions. A random review of three patients revealed at least 21 instances where

Medicaid paid for Vivitrol that was not dispensed to the recipient for whom it had been prescribed, the affidavit states.

Another nurse was arrested following an indictment by a grand jury on one count of Medicaid Fraud and one count of obtaining possession of a controlled substance by of fraud, misrepresentation or subterfuge. At the time the crimes are alleged to have been committed, she worked as an RN at a nursing center. The indictment charges her with obtaining Norco containing Hydrocodone, a schedule two controlled substance, from a patient in the center.

Another individual who worked for a doctor signed that doctor's name and that of certified nurse practitioners to prescription forms for herself and at least two family members between December 2013 and June 2014. The prescriptions included Norco, Alprazolam, Aldactone, Tramadol and Celexa, and were filled at multiple pharmacies.

At the time of her arrest, she had 5,550 pills of hydrocodone and 210 pills of Xanax, as well as 30 diet pills. Looking only at the opiate Hydrocodone, that equates to an estimated 30.8 pills that would be taken per day during the six-month period charged in the felony complaint if it were for personal use as she alleged.

Health care consumers need to identify these health care fraudsters and report them to attempt to salvage the health care system. People need to remember that he/she could receive a monetary reward for being a whistle blower.

Whistle blowers are people who expose unethical or illegal wrongdoing within companies by reporting it internally to superiors or externally to the media, government authorities, or specialized attorneys. They can be either current or past employees (insiders), or outside individuals who are familiar with the unlawful conduct, and are not required to be U.S. citizens. If you properly report Medicare fraud, you may be entitled to a significant whistleblower reward.

23. Physical Therapy Fraud

Physical therapy is an important modality that can be used to help manage your pain. A therapist will rehabilitate you following an injury. Your strength and range of motion will be evaluated and treated. Your doctor will refer you to a physical therapist if he or she feels that this modality can be of some benefit to you. Physical therapists are highly trained individuals who will obtain a medical history from you and perform an examination on you.

Your physical therapist will decide which treatment is best for you based on your overall health after an evaluation. Your physical therapist will emphasize to you that you yourself are a major component in your rehabilitation and in the management of your chronic pain. Your physical therapist also will train you to avoid future re-injury and/or a recurrence of your pain problems.

Your physical therapist will emphasize flexibility exercises for you and show you how to do them. You have to learn to be able to move your joints without stiffness and pain. Furthermore, your physical therapist will work with you on your endurance and strength. Most importantly, your pain will be addressed. In many instances, a reduction in stiffness in combination with increases in strength and endurance will significantly reduce your pain.

For example, if you have a history of angina, your therapist will not overly stress you during exercise-related treatments because this may cause an increase in your heart rate and cause you to have chest pain. If you have had surgery or have been involved in a motor vehicle accident, it is important that you tell your therapist while he or she is taking your history. Your therapist will need to become familiar with your pain history as well as your current pain complaints in order to formulate a treatment plan specific for you.

You should not be reluctant to give your therapist your age. Many conditions occur within certain age ranges. Osteoarthritis and osteoporosis are known to occur in an older population. Your therapist must know your occupation. If your job involves heavy physical labor, for example, you may be prone to overstress of your back muscles. Tell your therapist when the pain gets worse during the day or notify your therapist if you have increased pain with certain activities. With this information, your therapist can direct an appropriate therapy program for you.

If you have had a similar pain syndrome before your most current pain syndrome, again tell your therapist. If the intensity, duration, and frequency of your pain are increasing during therapy, your therapist may want to send you back to your doctor. This is an indication that you are becoming worse with respect to what is causing your pain and not from the physical therapy.

If your pain is worse during the morning and becomes progressively better during the day, this may be an indication that you have arthritis. Your therapist will need to know this information in order to prescribe the proper treatment for you. Providing a good medical history to your therapist will make it much easier for the therapist to prescribe the proper method of treatment for you.

If you are experiencing significant pain during your therapy, immediately notify your therapist and discontinue the treatment. One goal of physical therapy is to identify the cause of your pain with an attempt to treat the cause of your pain syndrome. In addition to rehabilitating you following your injury or illness, your physical therapist will attempt to correct any mechanical flaws in your body that could lead to further injury, such as your posture.

It has been shown that electricity can stimulate tissue growth and repair such as bone and is sometimes used by orthopedic surgeons to stimulate bone growth following bone surgery. Sometimes stimulators can be placed following orthopedic surgery to enhance bone growth. Theoretically, the electrical current should speed up your healing time. A popular electric current emitting device that is used frequently in pain medicine by conventional physicians, chiropractic physicians, and physical therapists is the transcutaneous electrical nerve stimulator (TENS).

Physical therapists can help you decrease your muscle tension. Your therapist also can educate you on how to decrease muscle tension yourself. Most muscle tension is related to the stress of everyday life. While flying on an airplane, for example, you may experience stress when the plane bounces around in turbulent weather. You may experience stress in your job if you have to make a presentation in front of a group. The muscles throughout your body naturally tense up when you are stressed.

The so-called "Rock Doc" who pleaded guilty to defrauding Medicare of $2.6 million through bogus physical therapy services has been sentenced to six years in prison. In addition to the billing fraud, this practitioner also admitted to illegally prescribing controlled substances and receiving kickbacks for referring patients for physical therapy, which was never done and has been ordered to repay Medicare about $1.65 million. The sentencing, which occurred, was reported in the Wall Street Journal and Miami Herald, among other outlets.

This health care provider was the subject of a 2010 WSJ front-page article that tracked nearly $1.2 million in payments from Medicare, mostly for "physical therapy" that was not provided by licensed physical therapists or not provided at all as mentioned. The family physician earned his nickname thanks in part to his high-profile lifestyle and punk appearance, complete with spiked blond hair.

Another case alleges that a physical therapist was the owner and operator of a physical therapy clinic. Patients would seek treatment at the clinic for minor injuries, generally sustained in car accidents. This clinic employed, a physical therapist, a physical therapy assistant; and an office manager. The indictment alleged that all off these employees conspired together to falsify patient treatment charts to reflect therapy that was either never given, or was performed by unlicensed personnel, including the clinic owner herself. The owner caused these fraudulent physical therapy claims to be submitted by mail to private insurance companies for payment. Various insurance companies paid more than $400,000 in bodily injury claims to the clinic and its "patients" during a two-year period, based on these fraudulent submissions.

In the next example, nothing about the clinic mentions at the money that is said to have flown there. But in 2012, according to federal data, $4.1 million from Medicare coursed through the billing office in a modest white house. In all, the practice treated around 1,950 Medicare patients that year. On average, it was paid by Medicare for 94 separate procedures for each one. That works out to about 183,000 treatments a year, 500 a day, 21 an hour. What makes those figures more remarkable, and raises eyebrows among medical experts, is that judging by Medicare billing records, one person did it all.

But physical therapy, it turns out, is a big recipient of national Medicare dollars and physical therapy in Brooklyn is among the biggest of all. Of the 10 physical therapists nationwide who were paid the most by Medicare in 2012, half listed Brooklyn's addresses, according to an analysis of Medicare billing data by The New York Times. Two others listed addresses on Long Island, one in Queens, and one each in California and Texas.

According to court documents in another case, a physical therapy assistant was paid beginning in June 2009 to falsify medical documentation, a home health agency owned by his alleged co-conspirators. This individual, a physical therapy assistant, pleaded guilty to creating evaluations, therapy revisit notes, and other medical documentation memorializing purported physical therapy for patients he did not see or treat.

According to court documents, an alleged co-conspirator instructed this individual on how to falsify medical documentation. This individual also signed therapy revisit notes as a physical therapy assistant for patients he did not see or treat and admitted to knowing that the documents he falsified and the documents he signed would be used to support false claims to Medicare for home-health services.

Another case involved a partner in a gym, which provided exercise, strength, conditioning and performance coaching services to students, faculty and staff at certain independent high schools in New Jersey. These conspirators developed a scheme to enrich themselves by billing their personal training sessions as physical therapy services covered by health insurance even though no one at the gym was a physical therapist.

The co-conspirators would ask clients for their health insurance in-formation and then lie to the insurance companies, indicating that the gym provided physical therapy. Some clients came to the gym with a doctor's prescription for physical therapy, and the gym would treat those individuals under the prescription and then bill the insurers. For other clients who had never seen a doctor. The physical therapy assistant made up his own diagnosis and then billed insurers as if he had provided physical therapy.

Another employee admitted that she hired an uncertified occupational therapy assistant, who fabricated and signed notes for occupational therapy patient visits that the assistant purported to perform. This employee the uncertified assistant for creating these fictitious patient visits notes and countersigned them. She also filled out patient discharge paperwork. She provided no services to the patients whose files she created and counter-signed. She was paid for each patient file that she created and knew that neither, she nor the uncertified occupational therapy assistant were providing occupational therapy services to the beneficiaries as stated in the falsified files.

In Los Angeles, authorities said court documents show clients who visited a rehabilitation facility and other related facilities sometimes received services like massage or acupuncture, which are not covered by Medicare, and were billed from practitioners not licensed to perform physical therapy, but received no covered services. In exchange for patient referrals, kickbacks were paid by "principals" at the facilities equal to about 55 percent of the reimbursement received from Medicare, the U.S. Attorney's office said.

In Florida, an indictment was made against a couple which stated that falsified patient records, and submitted fraudulent claims for services never provided, submitted claims by a therapist who wasn't enrolled as a Medicaid provider and submitted false claims for individual therapy that was actually performed in a group setting. This couple purportedly provided services to indigent or disabled patients and billed Medicaid for those services. They purportedly offered services to elderly people in assisted-living homes and billed Medicare. The couple agreed to forfeit $319,415, which is the total amount they collectively received from Medicare and Medicaid.

Some of the largest perpetrators of Medicare fraud are nursing homes. When engaging in Medicare fraud, nursing homes provide patients with services that they do not need, and bill Medicare for the reimbursements. In one particularly egregious case, a nursing home within in a national chain billed Medicare for physical therapy, occupational therapy, and speech therapy for a single patient all in the same day. Meanwhile, the patient, who was 92-years-old and very ill, died the next day.

The rise of for-profit nursing homes is proving tragic for some of the nation's most vulnerable people, resulting in a spike in waste, fraud and abuse charges brought by federal authorities, according to a new report. Seventy percent of nursing homes were operated on a for-profit basis in 2010, according to an audit by the Medicare Payment Advisory Commission, which counsels Congress. For-profit nursing homes perform better financially: Their profit margins from treating Medicare patients were 21 percent in 2010 compared with 10 percent for non-profit nursing-home companies, the commission reported.

Cases filed against the for-profit nursing homes by law enforcement and by families of patients who died allege that for-profit nursing-home companies pressure facility managers to minimize the number of employees and keep down their hours to save costs. At the same time, these firms pushed for patients to receive services they did not need, according to the allegations.

A Texas federal jury on Monday found that the CEO and two other top executives of a chain of physical therapy clinics focused on treating federal government employees committed health care fraud and money laundering, but acquitted a chiropractor who was allegedly in on the scheme. The jury deliberated for about 14 hours following a 16-day trial before finding the CEO, chief financial officer and vice president of the five-state chain of these clinics guilty of all counts related to their alleged scheme to defraud the government under the Federal Employees Compensation Act, according to court records and the U.S. Department of Justice. Prosecutors alleged the executives directed chiropractors at four of their clinics to submit $9.6 million worth of false and fraudulent claims under FECA for services that weren't provided to patients.

Health care consumers need to identify these health care fraudsters and report them to attempt to salvage the health care system. People need to remember that he/she could receive a monetary reward for being a whistle blower.

Whistle blowers are people who expose unethical or illegal wrongdoing within companies by reporting it internally to superiors or externally to the media, government authorities, or specialized attorneys. They can be either current or past employees (insiders), or outside individuals who are familiar with the unlawful conduct, and are not required to be U.S. citizens. If you properly report Medicare fraud, you may be entitled to a significant whistleblower reward.

24. Occupational Therapy Fraud

Occupational therapy is the use of assessment and intervention to develop, recover, or maintain the meaningful activities, or occupations, of individuals, groups, or communities. It is an allied health profession performed by occupational therapists. These therapists often work with people with disabilities, injuries, or impairments.

According to the plea documents, an occupational therapist who worked at a physical therapy clinic which purported to provide physical and occupational therapy services to patients. In 2005, this therapist was hired by a clinic to create and sign falsified occupational therapy files. This therapist created patient evaluation forms for Medicare beneficiaries whom she had never met, seen or evaluated.

The therapist in question admitted that she hired an uncertified occupational therapy assistant, who fabricated and signed notes for occupational therapy patient visits that the assistant purported to perform. She paid the uncertified assistant for creating these fictitious patient visit notes and countersigned them. She also filled out patient discharge paperwork.

These individuals provided no services to the patients whose files she created and countersigned. The therapist was paid for each patient file that she created. She knew that neither, she nor the uncertified occupational therapy assistant was providing occupational therapy services to the beneficiaries as stated in the falsified files.

The therapist admitted that between approximately June 2005 and May 2007, she and her co-conspirators at the therapy clinic submitted or caused the submission of fraudulent claims to the Medicare program. She submitted or caused to be submitted approximately $897,512 in claims for occupational therapy services that were never rendered.

A federal judge gave an occupational therapist the green light to file a Whistle Blower law suit against the nation's largest nursing home operator and contract physical therapy company for submitting false Medicare and Medicaid claims for years. As part of a guilty plea, another occupational therapist admitted that he owned an occupational therapy clinic in California, but hid his ownership in the name of a "straw "or nominee owner in an effort to execute and conceal a fraudulent scheme. He admitted that as part of the scheme, he billed Medicare for occupational therapy services when no such services were provided to the Medicare beneficiaries.

Instead, the Medicare beneficiaries received acupuncture and massage services, which were not reimbursable by Medicare. He further admitted that he directed co-conspirator therapists to falsify medical records to make it appear as if the services billed had been actually provided and funneled 87 percent of the proceeds from Medicare to himself.

Among the cases involving therapy were five individuals in New York charged with illegal activities involving some $86 million in fraudulent physical therapy and occupational therapy claims. According to a press release, the individuals under indictment in this case filled a network of Brooklyn's clinics that they controlled with patients by paying bribes and kickbacks. Once at the clinics, these patients were subjected to medically unnecessary therapy. The defendants are alleged to have used over a dozen shell companies to launder the money they received from Medicare. The suit charges that this clinic established internal guidelines requiring the delivery of expensive skilled rehabilitation therapies such as physical, occupational, or speech therapies that were not medically reasonable or necessary.

More specifically, this clinic allegedly set and closely monitored adherence to excessive corporate goals for the provision of "Ultra High" patient therapies, which offer the highest level of allowable Medicare reimbursement rates, regardless of the patient's medical condition. Additionally, the clinic also established length of stay targets for Medicare patients that closely paralleled the allowable time period for benefit coverage.

The documents also reveal stories of patients, like a 92-year-old dying of metastatic cancer. Two days before his death, he was spitting out blood. The clinic therapists, however, still recorded 48 minutes of physical therapy, 47 minutes of occupational therapy, and 30 minutes of speech therapy that very day.

In her plea a licensed occupational therapist, admitted that she began working in approximately September 2005 as a contract therapist for a co-conspirator who entered a guilty plea in the same case in September. An accomplice owned and controlled several companies operating in the Detroit area that claimed to provide physical and occupational therapy services to Medicare beneficiaries. The therapist admitted that she, the clinic owner, and others created fictitious therapy files appearing to document occupational therapy services provided to Medicare beneficiaries, when, in fact, no such services had been provided. According to court documents, the fictitious services reflected in the files were billed to Medicare through sham Medicare providers controlled by the co-conspirators.

The occupational therapist admitted that her role in creating the fictitious therapy files was to sign documents and progress notes indicating she had provided occupational therapy services to particular Medicare beneficiaries, when, in fact she had not. She was paid between $90 and $110 by the clinic owner per file that she falsified in this manner.

She also admitted that in the course of the arrangement charged under the indictment, she signed approximately 544 fictitious occupational therapy files, falsely indicating she had provided occupational therapy services to Medicare beneficiaries. She admitted she knew that the files she helped falsify were used to justify fraudulent billings to Medicare.

Another individual worked at a therapy center in Minnesota for three years. According to court documents, she oversaw the time clients were on exercise machines in a wellness center, without supervision. She says those records were used by the clinic owner to bill the therapy center for occupational therapy and physical therapy services. The therapy center, then would bill Medicare or Medicaid.

Additionally, "in some instances, this individual witnessed the instituitions physical therapists negotiating over who would get to claim her time as their own that day in order to meet the clinic's established individual productivity goals," court records state. After this therapist went to work for another clinic, she said what she had seen at her previous clinic prompted her in filing the lawsuit in 2008. This therapist "alleged the time, place and manner of the fraud and identified 41 specific incidents of false billing," and provided enough facts for the case to move to discovery.

A USA TODAY analysis reveals that some of Medicare's top-earning specialists are in the New York City borough and sharing thousands of Medicare patients in volumes much higher than the norm. In hundreds of cases, patients have seen several pain specialists on the same day, shuffling between therapists who have billed Medicare for tens of thousands of procedures. In one case, a chiropractor and an occupational therapist saw the same patients on the same day more than 11,000 times in 18 months.

These high-earning occupational therapists, chiropractors and physical therapists have given Brooklyn an unusual distinction that it either has the most damaged group of elderly and disabled patients in the country or perhaps a problem with fraud. According to the plea documents, an uncertified occupational therapy assistant worked for a physical therapy clinic which alleged to provide physical and occupational therapy services. In 2005, this individual was hired by a co-defendant to create and sign falsified occupational therapy files for this therapy clinic, which was owned and operated by two co-defendants.

This person purported to be a certified occupational therapy assistant and fabricated and signed patient notes for occupational therapy services that she claimed she had provided. In fact, the services were never provided. Furthermore, as an unsupervised and uncertified assistant, she was not permitted to perform the occupational therapy services.

A Pompano Beach occupational therapist that used swimming to treat stroke victims and other patients has been arrested on a charge of falsely billing Medicare by $586,000, federal court documents show. This individual who owned the aquatic therapy services, billed for more hours of therapy than she provided, for individual therapy when patients were in group sessions, and for a therapist's time when lesser-trained employees were present, according to documents filed Tuesday. She put patients in pools to help them recover lost physical abilities. She filed phony bills from 2008 through last year.

The therapist admitted that between approximately June 2005 and May 2007, she and her co-conspirators at the therapy clinic submitted or caused the submission of fraudulent claims to the Medicare program. She submitted or caused to be submitted approximately $897,512 in claims for occupational therapy services that were never rendered. As part of a guilty plea, an occupational therapist admitted that he owned an occupational therapy clinic in California, but hid his ownership in the name of a "straw "or nominee owner in an effort to execute and conceal a fraudulent scheme. He admitted that as part of the scheme, he billed Medicare for occupational therapy services when no such services were provided to the Medicare beneficiaries.

Instead, the Medicare beneficiaries received acupuncture and massage services, which were not reimbursable by Medicare. He further admitted that he directed co-conspirator therapists to falsify medical records to make it appear as if the services billed had been actually provided and funneled 87 percent of the proceeds from Medicare to himself.

Among the cases, involving therapy were five individuals in New York charged with illegal activities involving some $86 million in fraudulent physical therapy and occupational therapy claims. According to a press release, the individuals under indictment in this case filled a network of Brooklyn's clinics that they controlled with patients by paying bribes and kickbacks. Once at the clinics, these patients were subjected to medically unnecessary therapy. The defendants are alleged to have used over a dozen shell companies to launder the money they received from Medicare.

The suit charges that this clinic established internal guidelines requiring the delivery of expensive skilled rehabilitation therapies such as physical, occupational, or speech therapies that were not medically reasonable or necessary. More specifically, this clinic allegedly set and closely monitored adherence to excessive corporate goals for the provision of "Ultra High" patient therapies, which offer the highest level of allowable Medicare reimbursement rates, regardless of the patient's medical condition. Additionally, the clinic also established length of stay targets for Medicare patients that closely paralleled the allowable time period for benefit coverage.

The documents also reveal stories of patients, like a 92-year-old dying of metastatic cancer. Two days before his death, he was expelling out blood. The clinic therapists, however, still recorded 48 minutes of physical therapy, 47 minutes of occupational therapy, and 30 minutes of speech therapy that very day.

In her plea a licensed occupational therapist, admitted that she began working in approximately September 2005 as a contract therapist for the co-conspirator who entered a guilty plea in the same case in September. An accomplice owned and controlled several companies operating in the Detroit area that claimed to provide physical and occupational therapy services to Medicare beneficiaries. The therapist admitted that she, the clinic owner, and others created fictitious therapy files appearing to document occupational therapy services provided to Medicare beneficiaries, when in fact no such services had been provided. According to court documents, the fictitious services reflected in the files were billed to Medicare through sham Medicare providers controlled by the co-conspirators.

The occupational therapist admitted that her role in creating the fictitious therapy files was to sign documents and progress notes indicating she had provided occupational therapy services to particular Medicare beneficiaries, when in fact she had not. She was paid between $90 and $110 by the clinic owner per file that she falsified in this manner.

She also admitted that in the course of the arrangement charged in the indictment, she signed approximately 544 fictitious occupational therapy files, falsely indicating she had provided occupational therapy services to Medicare beneficiaries. She admitted she knew that the files she helped falsify were used to justify fraudulent billings to Medicare.

Another individual worked at a therapy center in Minnesota for three years. According to court documents, she oversaw the time clients were on exercise machines in a wellness center, without supervision. She says those records were used by the clinic owner to bill the therapy center for occupational therapy and physical therapy services. The therapy center, then would bill Medicare or Medicaid.

Additionally, in some instances, the occupational therapist witnessed the physical therapy, therapists negotiating over who would get to claim the occupational therapist's time as their own that day in order to meet clinic established individual productivity goals, court records state. After the occupational therapist went to work for another clinic, she said what she had seen at her previous clinic, and other employees joined her in filing her lawsuit.

A USA TODAY analysis revealed that some of Medicare's top-earning specialists are in the New York City borough and sharing thousands of Medicare patients in volumes much higher than the norm. In hundreds of cases, patients have seen several pain specialists on the same day, shuffling between therapists who have billed Medicare for tens of thousands of procedures. In one case, a chiropractor and an occupational therapist saw the same patients on the same day more than 11,000 times in 18 months.

These high-earning occupational therapists, chiropractors and physical therapists have given Brooklyn an unusual distinction that it either has the most damaged group of elderly and disabled patients in the country or perhaps a problem with fraud. According to the plea documents, an uncertified occupational therapy assistant worked for a physical therapy clinic which alleged to provide physical and occupational therapy services. In 2005, this individual was hired by a co-defendant to create and sign falsified occupational therapy files for this therapy clinic, which was owned and operated by two co-defendants.

This person purported to be a certified occupational therapy assistant and fabricated and signed patient notes for occupational therapy services that she claimed she had provided. In fact, the services were never provided. Furthermore, as an unsupervised and uncertified assistant, she was not permitted to perform the occupational therapy services.

Another occupational group was charged with alleged violations, which included: Placing patients in the highest-possible reimbursement levels, regardless of determinations made through patient evaluation, Boosting the amount of reported therapy during assessment reference periods" and then providing less therapy to those patients outside of those reference periods, Scheduling and reporting the provision of therapy, even after the patients' therapist had recommended discharge, Shifting minutes of planned therapy among disciplines to ensure targeted therapy reimbursement levels were achieved, regardless of the clinical need for therapy, Providing higher amounts of therapy near the end of a therapy measurement period to maximize payment, Reporting time spent on initial evaluation as therapy time rather than evaluation time, Reporting that skilled therapy had been provided when in fact the patients were asleep or otherwise unable to undergo or benefit from skilled therapy and Reporting estimated or rounded minutes of therapy rather than actual minutes provided.

Health care consumers need to identify these health care fraudsters and report them to attempt to salvage the health care system. People need to remember that he/she could receive a monetary reward for being a whistle blower.

Whistle blowers are people who expose unethical or illegal wrongdoing within companies by reporting it internally to superiors or externally to the media, government authorities, or specialized attorneys. They can be either current or past employees (insiders), or

outside individuals who are familiar with the unlawful conduct, and are not required to be U.S. citizens. If you properly report Medicare fraud, you may be entitled to a significant whistleblower reward.

25. Allergist Fraud

An allergist/immunologist is a physician trained to prevent, diagnose, manage, and treat allergic disease. As a result of extensive study and training, allergists/immunologists are highly qualified to manage immune system disorders such as allergies, asthma, inherited immunodeficiency diseases, and autoimmune diseases.

Some allergy problems such as a mild case of hay fever may not need any treatment. Sometimes allergies can be controlled with the occasional use of an over-the-counter medication. However, often allergies can interfere with day-to-day activities or decrease the quality of life. Allergies can even be life threatening.

An allergist is a physician who specializes in the diagnosis and treatment of asthma and other allergic diseases. The allergist is specially trained to identify the factors that trigger asthma or allergies. Allergists help people treat or prevent their allergy problems. After earning a medical degree, the allergist completes a three-year residency-training program in either internal medicine or pediatrics. Next the allergist completes two or three more years of study within the field of allergy and immunology.

One of the marvels of the human body is that it can defend itself against harmful invaders such as viruses or bacteria. However, sometimes the defenses are too aggressive and harmless substances such as dust, molds or pollen are mistakenly identified as dangerous. The immune system then rallies its defenses, which include several chemicals to attack and destroy the supposed enemy. In the process, some unpleasant and, in extreme cases, life-threatening symptoms may be experienced in the allergy-prone individual.

Many different types of doctors treat allergies and sinus problems. And if you have sinus problems, you should go to an ear, nose and throat board certified otolaryngologist who specializes in the treatment of sinus problems and allergies. If you have skin problems, you may also need to see a dermatologist from the itchy skin. If your eyes itch or burn from the allergies, we may have to send you to an ophthalmologist or an eye doctor, but it should really be a team of doctors, including a board-certified allergist who treats your sinus problems and your allergies and makes sure that together all the doctors have given you the best that they will all have to give you the best possible result possible.

Since the underlying cause of sinus disease and related symptoms is frequently allergy, an allergist should always be seen first. If your allergist suspects structural problems in combination with allergic symptoms, he will gladly guide you to an ENT for proper care.

Allergy testing and immunotherapy schemes continue to pop up in primary care practices across the country, exposing patients and families to substandard diagnosis and treatment as well as raising the potential for fraudulent billing. However, there are deceptions too and here is how to recognize the signs of fraud.

Primary care offices enter into agreements with third-party companies whereby a "certified allergy specialist" tests patients and recommends treatment. Patients are shuffled in for environmental and/or food allergy testing, and then offered immunotherapy, which may include either allergy shots or sublingual immunotherapy (SLIT) in which drops of the allergen are placed under the tongue. Many patients are unaware that SLIT is not currently approved and, therefore, not typically reimbursable by insurance.

Meanwhile, patients are unaware that these "certified allergy specialists" are not formally trained allergists. Many treatments recommended are inconsistent with established standards of practice designed to protect you as the patient. Jim Wallen, an expert in allergy extract testing and immunotherapy states, "Because drops are not FDA-approved, they are typically not reimbursable by health insurance. However, many primary care practices, some unknowingly, bill insurance companies.

This is just one example of insurance billing fraud. Others include maximizing the number of allergens tested in order to maximize reimbursement; giving extremely low doses to avoid reactions, although reimbursement remains the same; and treating with a universal stock mix that contains many allergens a patient is not allergic to." Many of these "certified allergy specialists" have no previous medical experience whatsoever and are given quotas for the number of patients they must test and put on allergy shots or risk losing their job.

Many dubious practitioners claim that food allergies may be responsible for virtually any symptom a person can have. In support of this claim which is false they administer various tests purported to identify offending foods. Claims of this type may seem credible because about 25% of people think they are allergic to foods. However, scientific studies have found that only about 6% of children and 1-2% of adults actually have a food allergy, and most people with food allergies are allergic to less than four foods.

The most notorious such test was cytotoxic testing, which was promoted during the early 1980s by storefront clinics, laboratories, nutrition consultants, chiropractors, and medical doctors. Advocates claimed it could determine sensitivity to food, which they blamed for asthma, arthritis, constipation, diarrhea, hypertension, obesity, stomach disorders, and many other conditions. However, controlled studies never demonstrated reliability, and some studies found it highly unreliable.

For example, one study found that white cells from allergic patients reacted no differently when exposed to substances known to produce symptoms than when exposed to substances to which the patients were not sensitive. Government regulatory actions and unfavorable publicity have almost driven cytotoxic testing from the health marketplace. However, a few practitioners still perform it, and many use similar "food sensitivity" tests.

The correct way to assess a suspected food allergy or intolerance is to begin with a careful record of food intake and symptoms over a period of several weeks. Symptoms such as swollen lips or eyes, hives, or skin rash may be allergy-related, particularly if they occur within a few minutes (up to two hours) after eating. Diarrhea may be related to food intolerance. Vague symptoms such as dizziness, weakness, or fatigue are unlikely to be food-related.

The history-taking procedure should note the suspected foods, the amounts consumed, the length of time between ingestion and symptoms, whether there is a consistent pattern of symptoms after the food is consumed, and several other factors. Although nearly any food can cause an allergic reaction, a few foods account for about 90% of reactions. Among adults, these foods are peanuts, nuts, fish, and shellfish. Among children, they are eggs, milk, peanuts, soy, and wheat.

Proper medical evaluation done best by an allergist will include a careful review of your history and skin testing with food extracts (using a prick or puncture technique) to see whether an allergic mechanism is involved in your symptoms. In cases where skin testing might be dangerous, a radioactive allergy sensitivity test (RAST) may be appropriate. The RAST is a laboratory test in which the technician mixes a sample of the patient's blood with various food extracts to see whether antibodies to food proteins are present in the blood. It is not as reliable as skin testing and is more expensive. A negative prick or RAST test indicates a low probability of allergy to the test substance. Positive tests, however, have much less predictive value.

The FBI raided one of three target locations, executing search warrants. The feds wouldn't comment on the investigation, but Strickland heard plenty from some of the clinic patients. They gave blood and expected a readout on potential allergies, all at no cost to them. They received no results, but their insurance company received multiple bills.

"There's two other dates on there like we're being treated for allergies, and we didn't get treated. We didn't get anything," she said. The form shows Blue Cross was billed for three allergy treatments apiece. Each one was $3,600. Blue Cross actually paid out a little more than $2,000.

According to court documents, individuals who operated a California clinic, as a Medicare-billing mill. A physician admitted that he set up the clinic and found a doctor to act as the official physician of record. However, the physician acknowledged, the doctor served primarily as a "front" so that the office could use his Medicare billing number to submit Medicare claims.

The individual in question further admitted that he recruited and paid "cappers," individuals whose sole task was to find senior citizens in El Centro and convince them to go to the clinic. In exchange for providing their Medicare beneficiary numbers, the senior citizens received a free pair of shoes and/or a free buffet lunch. Once they arrived at the clinic, the beneficiaries were subject to a pre-determined gauntlet of tests, which were not based on the patient's medical needs and were provided without proper supervision by a physician. In some cases, the clinic billed Medicare although the tests were not provided at all.

"This defendant had no regard for the medical needs or well-being of patients," said U.S. Attorney Laura Duffy. "He exploited vulnerable seniors—even giving them unnecessary tests without a doctor's approval in order to get rich quick on the backs of taxpayers."

Many of the tests that the Clinic claimed to have administered to beneficiaries required either that a physician administer the test or that a physician be within the Clinic during testing. On over 800 occasions, the Clinic billed Medicare for these tests despite cell phone location records showing that the doctor was not in Imperial County at all during the times these tests were allegedly administered. The Clinic also submitted reimbursement from Medicare for allergy tests despite evidence showing that these tests were never performed in the Clinic by a doctor or anyone else.

Hundreds of people seeking allergy treatment were scammed into believing they were getting free tests in a scheme that cost insurance companies more than $1.5 million and put patients' health at risk. Federal prosecutors have charged. On Thursday morning, federal agents arrested a 49-year-old nurse from Harwood Heights, and another individual. Eight other people, including four doctors, also were charged in the alleged scheme. One doctor was accused of leading the scam through a group of companies he operated as the American Institute of Allergy, which allegedly charged patients' insurance companies for tests it advertised as free.

Patients were promised free blood tests while providing information about their health insurance to institute employees. Their blood was taken but wasn't submitted for testing until their insurance companies agreed to foot the bill, the indictment charged. At times, tests were delayed so long that blood samples deteriorated, making results unreliable; prosecutors charged. The alleged scheme began in 2000 and continued until early this year.

During that time, patients who tested positive for allergies were prescribed allergy shots, often without being evaluated by a doctor, prosecutors charged. In many cases, untrained employees of the allergy institute gave patients the shots under unsanitary conditions; the indictment charged. Moreover, patients frequently weren't warned of significant health risks they could face from the shots, prosecutors alleged.

Today they have more ways than ever to peddle their wares. In addition to TV, radio, magazines, newspapers, infomercials, mail, and even word-of-mouth, they now can use the Internet websites offer miracle cures; emails tell stories of overnight magic. Sadly, older people are often the target for such scams. In fact, a government study found that most victims of health care fraud are over age 65. The problem is serious. Unproven remedies may be harmful. They may also waste money. And, sometimes, using these remedies keeps people from getting the medical treatment they need.

AllergiCare Relief Centers are a chain of franchises started by a man who is not listed as having an MD or any other title. They offer diagnosis of allergies by biofeedback and treatment of allergies by laser acupuncture. They admit that the method is not backed by any science, and they claim that what they are doing is not medical treatment.

The practice of chiropractic does not include the treatment of hypersensitivity to foods, medications, environmental allergens, or venoms, (b) prohibit a chiropractor from advertising the ability to treat these conditions, and (c) specify that violating these provisions constitutes a cause for discipline by the State Board of Chiropractic Examiners. Although many chiropractors suggest that spinal manipulation can benefit people with allergies, there is no logical reason to believe that. The most definitive survey of chiropractic studies related to allergy was published in 2004.

Many of the claims of chiropractic success in asthma have been primarily based upon anecdotal evidence or uncontrolled case studies. Three recently reported randomized controlled studies showed benefit in subjective measures, such as quality of life, symptoms, and bronchodilator use; however, the differences were not statistically significant between controls and treated groups. There were no significant changes in any objective lung function measures. There is currently no evidence to support the use of chiropractic spinal manipulative therapy as a primary treatment for asthma or allergy.

Health care consumers need to identify these health care fraudsters and report them to attempt to salvage the health care system. People need to remember that he/she could receive a monetary reward for being a whistle blower.

Whistle blowers are people who expose unethical or illegal wrongdoing within companies by reporting it internally to superiors or externally to the media, government authorities, or specialized attorneys. They can be either current or past employees (insiders), or outside individuals who are familiar with the unlawful conduct, and are not required to be U.S. citizens. If you properly report Medicare fraud, you may be entitled to a significant whistleblower reward.

26. Anesthesia Fraud

According to Wikipedia, anesthesiologists provide medical care to patients in many different ways. They provide care during preoperative evaluation, in consultation with the surgical team, and assist physicians in the creation of a plan for anesthetic intervention tailored for each individual patient. Anesthesiologists often provide more intensive care techniques such as assistance with airway management, intraoperative life support and provision of pain control, intraoperative diagnostic stabilization, and proper postoperative management of patients.

Anesthesiology fraud usually involves fraud in billing. What is the Medicare billing requirement when an anesthesiologist bills for the services of resident, AA, or CRNA? Insurance allows anesthesiologists to bill for the services of CRNA, residents, and AA. Anesthesiologists are allowed to provide medical direction for up to four concurrent cases provided several conditions are met and documented.

The anesthesiologist in order to charge for services must: 1. Perform the pre-anesthetic examination and evaluation of the patient.2. Prescribe the anesthetic plan. 3. Personally participate in induction, emergence and other aspects of the anesthesia plan. 4. Any procedures not performed by the physician must be done by a qualified anesthesia provider. 5. Monitor the anesthesia administration at regular intervals. 6. Remain physically present and available for immediate diagnosis and treatment of emergencies. 7. Provide indicated post-operative anesthesia care. 8. Provide documentation in the anesthesia record of the above.

Completion and compliance with these regulations requires strict discipline in a fluid healthcare environment. A study in 2012 determined that even with a supervision ratio of 1:2 there were lapses in supervision. An indictment, of an anesthesiologist accused this doctor that he provided anesthesia services personally and through a company he founded. From approximately 2009-2010, this doctor practiced medicine at two Dallas hospitals.

The indictment alleged that during this time, he ran a scheme to defraud Blue Cross Blue Shield of Texas (BCBS), United Healthcare (UHC), and the Federal Employees Health Benefits Program (FEHBP) by submitting, or causing to be submitted, false and fraudulent claims for personally performing medical direction of anesthesia services for certified registered nurse anesthetists (CRNAs).

He falsely represented that he was "present for" these services when: 1) he was under anesthesia undergoing surgery himself; 2) he was flying on his private jet; 3) he was in another state; and 4) he was at another hospital several miles away. For example, this doctor submitted or caused to be submitted several claims representing he was present for and medically directing six patients at two different hospitals and was medically directing two patients while under anesthesia himself.

The indictment further alleges that the doctor also inflated the amount of time the procedures took and pre-signed patients' medical records representing the services were provided before the procedures even took place. In addition to personally creating false medical records and inflating anesthesia procedure time, and he directed others to do the same, representing he was present for procedures when he knew he was not. As part of his approximate 18-month-long fraud scheme, he billed BCBS, UHC, and the FEHBP more than $8 million, of which at least $5 million was fraudulent.

Between about January 2005 and February 2008, two anesthesiologists conspired to overcharge Medicare, Medicaid, and other private health insurance companies at the Endoscopy Center of Southern Nevada by significantly overstating the amount of time the certified registered nurse anesthetists spent with patients on a given procedure.

These doctors created a separate company, owned by one of them to handle the billing for the anesthesia services. This company received approximately nine percent of all money collected for anesthesia services rendered at the endoscopy center. These doctors imposed intense pressure on the endoscopy center employees to schedule and treat as many patients as possible in a day, and instructed the nurse anesthetists to overstate in their records the amount of time they spent on the anesthesia procedures.

These anesthesiologists also instructed the office staff to rely on the false anesthesia records when preparing the claims for reimbursement, which were sent to Medicare, Medicaid and the insurance companies. The plea agreement states that Rushing received approximately $1.3 million as her share of the inflated anesthesia billing scheme.

A university paid $1.2 million to resolve allegations that it had been allowing Certified Registered Nurse Anesthetists or residents to administer anesthesia without a supervisory anesthesiologist being either present or available. Lawyers for the whistle blower filed a suit stating that even when the supervisor was not present, the hospital filled out records – in advance of the surgery, even to make it look like the surgeon was there. The hospital then billed for the higher rate it was entitled to charge if the anesthesiologists directly supervised the medical procedures. The California Board of Regents paid the United States government in order to resolve the allegations that the university had overcharged Medicare by this practice.

There are a shocking number of cries about fraud by anesthesiologists and anesthesia groups far and away more than for any other type of Medicare fraud, Medicaid fraud or government contract procurement fraud. Because of the way the anesthesia field is set up, almost all of these cases all revolve about the question of supervision. Certainly, most people who go into the hospital are under the impression that a doctor is administering their anesthesia. In fact, frequently a nurse anesthetist is administering the anesthesia. A nurse anesthetist does have some specialized training in anesthesia, but is not a M.D.

Under Medicare's rules, an anesthesiologist can bill Medicare the most if he or she personally performs the anesthesia. However, the anesthesiologist also can bill for "medically directing" anesthetists who actually perform the procedures. The Medicare rules require several conditions to prove that the anesthesiologist actually is doing the supervising. For example, the anesthesiologist has to be present at certain; key points in the procedure, and has to be on call to help.

The anesthesiologists only can request reimbursement for four or fewer anesthesiology procedures at the same time. The point of all of these rules, of course, is to make sure that the doctor is really involved in and supervising the work being done on patients. If the anesthesiologist is not as involved in the supervision, he still can bill Medicare if he supervises the anesthetists less closely, but in that case, he must expect a lower rate for his work in "medically supervising" the process.

An anesthesiologist practicing in Bloomington, Indiana has been charged with healthcare fraud, healthcare fraud resulting in serious bodily injury and 11 counts of unlawful drug distribution. The indictment alleges this doctor required patients to undergo medically unnecessary injection procedures, so they could receive narcotic controlled substance prescriptions; that the injection procedures were performed with a frequency and pattern not medically necessary and outside the bounds of medical practice and not for a legitimate medical purpose.

Furthermore, the doctor prescribed controlled substances as part of a scheme to defraud healthcare benefit programs by providing drug-dependent patients with controlled substances to encourage patients to submit to unwanted and unnecessary injection procedures and other services; and that he caused patients to become dependent on medically unnecessary procedures.

Medicare and state insurance programs pay only for services that are "reasonable and necessary for the diagnosis or treatment of illness or injury." In submitting claims to Medicare for reimbursement, healthcare providers "certify" that they have complied with relevant and "material" regulations governing the services they provide.

The whistle blower who filed suit against an anesthesiologist claimed that the healthcare provider was using "under-qualified" professionals to perform anesthesia, was "up-charging" the government, and used "kickbacks" to drum-up business.

A chiropractor/anesthesiologist scheme scammed various private insurance companies to pay millions of dollars on behalf of patients who underwent an experimental form of manipulation under anesthesia at a surgical center. Manipulation under anesthesia is an aggressive form of therapy typically reserved for patients who failed with conservative chiropractic care. There were serious risks associated with it, according to the indictment.

Because of the pain involved during manipulation, patients were put under conscious sedation and it was recognized as a surgical procedure. It was not performed in an office setting but rather an outpatient surgical facility and typically generated three types of insurance claims for professional fees, facility fees and fees for anesthesia services, according to the indictment.

Beginning in 2008, an anesthesiologist and others began marketing a surgical center and the manipulation under anesthesia procedure to chiropractors in Ohio, typically at restaurants in downtown Cleveland or the Youngstown area. In return for referring patients to a particular surgical center for the manipulation under anesthesia procedure, chiropractors were paid a flat fee of $4,000 per patient referred for a three-day session of procedures. Patients were advised they would not have to pay anything for the procedure, according to the indictment.

The defendants disregarded diagnoses, used false diagnoses, submitted false billing claims, represented that procedures were performed by osteopathic and medical doctors when, in reality, they were performed by osteopathic doctors and chiropractors, waived patients' required co-payments and deductibles, and took other steps as part of the criminal conspiracy. This took place between 2007 and 2010, according to the indictment. Prosecutors are also seeking to seize property derived from the criminal conspiracy, including two properties in Boca Raton, FL., a Royal Oak Offshore Chronograph watch and 4.18-karat diamond stud earrings, as well as money, according to the indictment.

One of California's largest health care givers, fraudulently charged insurers up to hundreds of millions of dollars over the past decade for anesthesia services that in some cases weren't even provided. The alleged health care fraud by a doctor includes billing for services never provided to patients, submitting claims for services and testing that were not medically necessary, billing for tests and equipment provided by an outside laboratory vendor, and "up coding,"" or submitting claims for procedures and tests with higher reimbursement codes than the actual procedures or tests performed. The alleged fraudulent claims were submitted to the Delaware Medicaid program, as well as to Medicare and third-party private insurers.

Health care consumers need to identify these health care fraudsters and report them to attempt to salvage the health care system. People need to remember that he/she could receive a monetary reward for being a whistle blower.

Whistle blowers are people who expose unethical or illegal wrongdoing within companies by reporting it internally to superiors or externally to the media, government authorities, or specialized attorneys. They can be either current or past employees (insiders), or outside individuals who are familiar with the unlawful conduct, and are

not required to be U.S. citizens. If you properly report Medicare fraud, you may be entitled to a significant whistleblower reward.

27. Cosmetic Surgery Fraud

Plastic surgery is a surgical specialty involving the restoration, reconstruction, or alteration of the human body. It includes cosmetic or aesthetic surgery, reconstructive surgery, craniofacial surgery, hand surgery, microsurgery, and the treatment of burns. Every year, millions of Americans elect to have cosmetic surgery. In response to this growing demand, numerous doctors now widely advertise their services in this area of medical expertise. Most surgeons performing cosmetic surgery are qualified; however, beware of inexperienced and insufficiently trained doctors who are attracted to cosmetic surgery because of the millions of dollars spent by consumers each year on this service.

Cosmetic surgery is popular. This fact causes some people to create their own make-believe medical experience and victimize innocent people. Recent studies show that most of the victims of unlicensed cosmetic surgery are everyday people, from those who are struggling to make ends meet to the considerably well-off looking on ways to improve their body while saving money. There is an increasing number of Americans that fall victim to empty promises given by opportunists. The fact is that more people are more concerned about the surgery result and cost of the surgery rather than the credentials and experience of the doctor. In this time of crisis, people are becoming more frugal but less careful.

Police are trying to track down an identity theft suspect who may now be exhibiting $10,000 in stolen breast implants. According to police, a female used an Illinois woman's identity to open a line of credit at a plastic surgery clinic. The 20-year-old allegedly used the account to get breast implants, liposuction, lip injections, etc. The cost for the procedures was more than $11,000.

There are several recorded cases of fraudulent cosmetic surgery procedures. One is a San Jose couple who were accused of performing at least nine botched surgeries without a license. Their surgeries were mostly performed in secrecy and in the couple's kitchen, which was considered filthy even by non-surgical standards. More horrifyingly, the couple used everyday kitchen utensils and instruments to perform some of the most complicated cosmetic surgery procedure, including tummy tucks, liposuction and breast augmentation.

The first thing a patient must do is to check if a doctor is board-certified. A doctor's certification is the best indicator of his or her experience and training in a specific surgical or medical expertise. However, you should also know what certification you are looking for in order to be completely sure. What you must look for is the ABPS or the American Board of Plastic Surgery certification. This certification is the only recognized board by the ABMS or the American Board of Medical Specialties.

Rhinoplasty is the most common procedure that is fraudulently billed to health insurance. Surgeons typically charge for repair of a "deviated septum" and then bill for rhinoplasty as well. Most people have a deviated septum, but that doesn't mean that they need to be operated on. Only when the septum blocks airflow and interferes with breathing does it need surgery. If the septum is twisted, it may be operated on for cosmetic reasons.

Tummy tucks are also fraudulently billed to insurance. Insurance companies may approve the procedure for problems created by pregnancy, but most will no longer do so. In an attempt to gain insurance coverage, separation of the abdominal muscles is sometimes fraudulently called a hernia. As any general surgeon will attest, this is not a true hernia and should not be covered by insurance.

Upper eyelid surgery is another area for fraud. Surgeons fraudulently claim that the eyelid skin blocks vision. There have even been conspiracies between ophthalmologists who have documented impaired visual fields and plastic surgeons that have performed the insurance-covered eyelid lifts.

Even more scandalous are the surgeons who perform liposuction and bill insurance companies for excision of "multiple lipomas." Some even try to bill insurance for breast augmentations, claiming the surgery was a breast reconstruction. Florida police officials zeroed in on a crime ring. Over the course of time, 14 Central Florida women were arrested and over a dozen, people fell victim to identity theft. The plastic surgery was tummy tucks, breast implants, breast reductions, whatever you could get with plastic surgery; that's what they were getting done.

Officials are unsure about how the plastic surgeon obtained the victims' information, but upon receiving it, she was able to tap into their credit card accounts and charged a small fee to people looking to get procedures done. In some instances, medical offices were able to spot the fraud before moving forward with the procedures. According to the police report, the plastic surgeon's cell phone number was used to call a credit card company over 300 times in less than a year. The phone number was reportedly linked to 16 accounts under the credit card company. Herb said the crime ring was the plastic surgeon's "full-time job."

Two administrators of a midtown medical clinic were charged with mail fraud and accused in a scheme to perform plastic surgery on patients without a license in which insurance companies were billed at least $350,000, according to a complaint unsealed in Federal District Court in Manhattan. One of the administrators was arrested by agents of the Federal Bureau of Investigation. The agents also seized records from the clinic, which offers reconstructive and cosmetic surgery. In outlining the scheme, prosecutors described numerous cases in which an employee, who is not a doctor, performed such procedures as the removal of skin lesions, vein treatments and lip enlargements. The clinic then billed the insurance companies as if the procedures were carried out by one of two licensed physicians associated with the clinic.

In one case described in the complaint, the clinic submitted forms to insurers that said a doctor affiliated with the clinic had removed 18 skin lesions from one patient, for which the clinic billed the insurance company a total of $9,500. This is the second recent case to raise concerns about who is performing plastic surgery.

In an unrelated matter, New York health regulators assessed a fine of $66,000 in December against a teaching hospital for failing to supervise two senior residents who were caught performing inexpensive plastic surgery on weekends, without the supervision of senior doctors.

A female scammer pulled off the $7,500 heist at a plastic surgery clinic. The young woman, believed to be 19, filled out paperwork for the surgery using the fake ID and then received surgery. After the operation, the criminal paid for the procedure with a bogus credit card. She then strolled out of the center with her new plus-sized chest and hasn't been seen since, sources said. It took over a year and a half for a plastic surgery clinic to report fraud because the credit card company had to untangle the web of deceit spun by the top heavy larcenist, sources said. The rep said the procedure can be done in two to three hours. First, the patient undergoes a pre-op consultation and fills out paperwork that ultimately determines how much her breasts will be surgically enhanced. Then the plastic surgeon performs the operation. Afterward, the patient goes through a two-day recovery period. The cunning offender wasn't required to go back to the clinic for a post op consultation because it's optional.

Two women were sentenced to federal prison on Friday for a medical fraud scheme that billed health insurance programs for more than $71 million in unnecessary medical procedures. Prosecutors said two individuals in San Pedro ran a scheme out of a surgery center where they connected patients with free or discounted cosmetic surgeries, including tummy tucks, breast augmentation and liposuction in exchange for undergoing procedures they didn't need, such as endoscopies and colonoscopies.

Under the scam, marketers enticed patients to a surgery center for consultations in which they were told that they could receive free or discounted cosmetic surgeries if they underwent multiple, medically unnecessary procedures that would be billed to their union or PPO health care benefit program. Many of the fraudulent claims were submitted to the International Longshore and Warehouse Union and Operating Engineers Union health insurance plans. Prosecutors said the loss as a result of unnecessary medical procedures was at least $2.6 million, based upon a review of just some of the claims.

A 28-year-old woman charged with masterminding a scheme to use stolen identities to pay for tens of thousands of dollars of plastic surgery, and dental work has been convicted of fraud. She was arrested in January 2016 as part of an operation which netted more than a dozen other arrests. One female was the one who set up fraudulent accounts and lines of credit using stolen identities from at least 12 people. Police said the group of women involved in the scheme took advantage of the scheme to get everything from breast implants to gold teeth.

In all, medical businesses and credit companies were taken for nearly $200,000, investigators said. Detectives said most of the victims were between 20 and 24 years old. They started receiving bills in the mail saying they owed thousands of dollars in medical bills.

Workers at a dental clinic discovered that a woman using someone else's information to have cosmetic dentistry done and contacted police. On top of the dental work, the woman also got breast implants using stolen credit. Police said another woman had liposuction done with stolen credit information.

A St. Louis-area plastic surgeon faces sentencing in January after admitting in federal court to billing patients for procedures that were unnecessary or never performed. This surgeon pleaded guilty to one misdemeanor charge of false demand against the United States. His firm pleaded guilty to one felony count of health care fraud. Court documents claim that the plastic surgeon and the company fraudulently billed insurance providers and the government for claims of $1 million.

A Los Angeles resident filed a lawsuit in Los Angeles Superior Court alleging that her plastic surgeon, conspired with medical device manufacturer Allergan, Inc., to promote and use SERI surgical scaffold and Natrelle breast tissue expanders in her in an off-label, experimental manner without her knowledge. She has sued the doctor and his practice for medical negligence, breach of fiduciary duty, lack of informed consent and fraud. She sued Allergan for negligence, fraud, and failure to warn and is seeking punitive damages.

According to the complaint filed by a San Diego Attorney, the SERI surgical scaffold never received clearance by the FDA for use in breast reconstruction or with the Natrelle breast expanders. The complaint goes on to allege that the doctor had an extensive financial/research relationship with Allergan, with financial and research interests in the SERI and Natrelle products.

A plastic surgeon has acted as a speaker and "faculty member" for Allergan, and consulted on the use and marketing of Allergan products. The complaint alleges that the doctor was paid by Allergan to promote and use its products, and at the time he treated the patient; he was a principal investigator for an ongoing FDA-sanctioned clinical study regarding the use of the SERI scaffold with the Natrelle breast expanders in breast reconstruction surgery. The patient was unaware of the doctor's extensive relationship with Allergan or his financial and research interests in the SERI and Natrelle products.

Surgeons extensively rely on photographic communication for documenting surgical results, teaching and research, and obtaining informed consent from patients. With the advent of digital photography and widespread availability of sophisticated image manipulation software, the potential for committing digital fraud cannot be discounted.

Ten 'before' and 'after' plastic surgical photographs were selected, and a number of them were digitally enhanced using standard desktop software by a non-expert in digital photography. A panel of 10 consultant plastic surgeons was asked to judge which, if any of the images had been digitally manipulated.

Expert assessment had a sensitivity of only 12% in identifying digitally manipulated images. Digital fraud is easy to commit and difficult to detect. Furthermore, a number of inadvertent and simple image manipulation functions can also amount to misrepresentation. There may be scope for cooperation within editorial circles to set standards for the submission of digital photographs. Surgeons need also to be aware of the potential for misrepresentation of information through digital image manipulation and exercise caution in the communication of digital photographic information.

Health care consumers need to identify these health care fraudsters and report them to attempt to salvage the health care system. People need to remember that he/she could receive a monetary reward for being a whistle blower.

Whistle blowers are people who expose unethical or illegal wrongdoing within companies by reporting it internally to superiors or externally to the media, government authorities, or specialized attorneys. They can be either current or past employees (insiders), or outside individuals who are familiar with the unlawful conduct, and are not required to be U.S. citizens. If you properly report Medicare fraud, you may be entitled to a significant whistleblower reward.

28. Cardiology Fraud

Cardiology is a branch of medicine dealing with disorders of the heart as well as parts of the circulatory system. The field includes medical diagnosis and treatment of congenital heart defects, coronary artery disease, heart failure, valvular heart disease and electrophysiology. Physicians who specialize in this field of medicine are called cardiologists, a specialty of internal medicine. Pediatric cardiologists are pediatricians who specialize in cardiology. Physicians who specialize in cardiac surgery are called cardiothoracic surgeons or cardiac surgeons, a specialty of general surgery.

Interventional cardiology is a branch of cardiology that deals specifically with the catheter based treatment of structural heart diseases. Andreas Gruentzig is considered the father of interventional cardiology after the development of angioplasty by interventional radiologist Charles Dotter. A large number of procedures can be performed on the heart by catheterization. This most commonly involves the insertion of a sheath into the femoral artery (but, in practice, any large peripheral artery or vein) and cannulating the heart under X-ray visualization (most commonly fluoroscopy).

The main advantages of using the interventional cardiology or radiology approach are the avoidance of the scars and pain, and long post-operative recovery. Additionally, interventional cardiology procedure of primary angioplasty is now the gold standard of care for an acute myocardial infarction. It involves the extraction of clots from occluded coronary arteries and deployment of stents, and balloons through a small hole made in a major artery. Over utilization, abuse, and fraud within cardiac departments have been receiving a great deal of media attention lately, since the federal government continues to demand that physicians and hospitals demonstrate that the invasive and expensive care they provide results in improved outcomes for patients.

Recently, a number of high-profile cases have shed light on the widespread extent of questionable physician and hospital practices, thereby underlying the importance of transparency and unbiased peer review in order to ensure that the quality of care meets professionally recognized standards. Hospitals are now being forced to demonstrate that cardiology procedures meet strict medical necessity criteria and guidelines. The penalties for inappropriate reimbursement are steep, with some physicians facing suspension or jail time and some hospitals facing millions of dollars in fines in addition to ruined reputations.

A complaint accused a cardiologist of routinely performing unnecessary tests that brought a high Medicare payment. They include ultrasounds of blood flow in the legs, stress tests and Holter monitoring for the heart, and nuclear imaging. Records would be falsified to include symptoms that would justify these tests. Another complaint says the cardiologist performed unnecessary catheterizations of the heart, a procedure that can have life-threatening complications. Cardiac catheterization involves inserting a flexible tube into a blood vessel and snaking it to the heart, injecting radioactive dye and taking nuclear images to show whether the blood is flowing properly in the coronary arteries and within the heart itself. Some patients were also subjected to unnecessary catheterization of blood vessels in arms and legs, the complaint says.

The heart institute regularly billed for procedures that were not performed at all through "up coding,"" instructing billers to code for more expensive procedures than the ones actually done. Also the physician routinely waived the 20 percent co-payment that Medicare requires patients to pay, probably to keep patients from questioning why they were getting so many tests.

The cardiologist sometimes went ahead with heart catheterizations without first taking a history, examining the patient or checking labs. One patient died, because she needed referral to a heart surgeon but the cardiologist delayed it to put stents in her leg vessels. Over the course of the conspiracy, the doctor ordered and performed essentially the same battery of diagnostic tests for nearly all the patients he treated, regardless of their symptoms. He also instructed his non-physician employees to order and perform diagnostic tests for patients of other doctors working at his offices, even though he had not examined those patients and the other physicians had not ordered the unnecessary tests.

Most significantly, the doctor admitted that he falsified patient charts with fictitious and boilerplate symptoms and falsely diagnosed a majority of his Medicare and Medicaid patients with coronary artery disease and debilitating and inoperable angina. He also admitted to making the diagnoses to justify prescribing and administering an unnecessary treatment for those patients called enhanced external counter pulsation, or EECP. Katz even prescribed EECP treatments for some patients with contraindications for the treatment, therefore, subjecting those patients to a substantial risk of serious injury or death.

This cardiologist was so focused on illegal profits that he directed unlicensed and unqualified providers to treat his patients, ordered unnecessary tests, and cavalierly ordered treatments that could have caused patient harm. Ripping off the government and insurance companies is bad enough but risking patient health in the bargain is inexcusable."

Unnecessary stents, unneeded catheterizations, unnecessary imaging tests, and referrals for heart surgery that were not medically warranted those are among the charges against an Ohio cardiologist, whose 16-count indictment was unsealed in federal court last week. The unnecessary medical tests and procedures cost Medicare and other insurers at least $7.2 million, according to federal enforcement agencies. According to the indictment, the doctor's other fraudulent activities included: Performing unnecessary nuclear imaging, aortograms, renal angiograms, intravascular ultrasound, and other tests that were not medically warranted. Recording false nuclear stress test results to justify cardiac catheterizations. Performing cardiac catheterizations and falsely recording occlusions or severity of disease.

This doctor falsely recorded symptoms to justify tests and procedures. Ian example is inserting stents in asymptomatic patients who did not have evidence of 70% stenosis. Furthermore, he referred patients for heart surgery when there was no medical necessity for surgery and this doctor to bill for follow-up testing.

In order to attract additional patients to the doctor's practice and maintain existing patients, this doctor would and did provide Schedule II controlled substances, including oxycodone, to drug-seeking patients, in exchange for those patients undergoing unnecessary diagnostic tests and other Medical Procedures.

A heart patient said he was persuaded at age 25 to have unnecessary surgery for an implant cardiac defibrillator, or ICD, which is similar to a pacemaker. A second physician recommended against it, saying his condition could be controlled with medication, but the patient said the cardiologist scared him. "He put the fear of God in me," the patient exclaimed. "When you have a doctor, a person you trust, sitting there looking you in the eye, and you can run the risk of dying and you're 25 years old; it's pretty intimidating."

Another patient filed a lawsuit under the False Claims Act against a cardiologist clinic and its owner, cardiologist and against a hospital; all located in Michigan alleging medically inappropriate cardiology procedures. The evidence showed that the cardiologist ordered cardiac catheters for patients based on findings from nuclear stress tests that he improperly read as positive. The government found that three-quarters of these patients had no significant heart blockages, according to a statement from the U.S. Attorney's Office of Eastern District of Michigan.

Another cardiologist received $13.4 million over a period of five years (2002-2007) by billing Medicare for reimbursement of extensive cardiac care that was not, according to an U.S. Attorney, ever performed. The cardiologist allegedly performed Medicare Fraud by hiring individuals to falsify patient names, insurance data, and dates in order to bill $8.3 million to Medicare and $5.1 million to other insurers.

Prosecutors say that the cardiologist, performed unnecessary cardiac stent procedures, in hundreds of patients, as part of a scheme to defraud Medicare, Medicaid, and other insurers. This doctor is charged with one count of health care fraud and 26 counts of making false statements relating to health care matters. A grand jury in Ashland indicted the cardiologist on the charges. In the indictment, investigators allege the scheme lasted from at least July 2008, when he retired. During that time, he is accused of performing more stent placement procedures than any cardiologist in Kentucky, and at times, more than any cardiologist in the US. Prosecutors said he subjected thousands of patients to unnecessary and potentially life-threatening treatments as a result of phony diagnoses.

"After years of prominence in his field, another cardiologist will now be remembered for his record-setting fraud." The doctor was so focused on illegal profits that he directed unlicensed and unqualified providers to treat his patients, ordered unnecessary tests and cavalierly ordered treatments that could have caused patient harm. Ripping off the government and insurance companies is bad enough; risking patient health in the bargain is inexcusable," said the prosecuting attorney.

This cardiologist also admitted keeping his wife on his payroll, even though she did little or no work, so she would be eligible for quarter-million dollars in Social Security. According to documents filed in this case and statements made in court, between July 2006 and February, 2009, the doctor spent more than $6 million for advertising on Spanish-language television and radio stations. The ads attracted hundreds of patients to the heart clinic every day. From 2005 through 2012, Medicare and Medicaid paid the cardiologist more than $15.6 million just for his enhanced external counter pulsation treatments, most of which were fraudulent, according to court documents.

A nurse in Fort Pierce, Florida, came forward with allegations that at least one doctor at his facility had been performing phony cardiac surgeries on healthy patients. After filing a complaint with the hospital's chief ethics office, it was determined that a number of doctors and surgeons within the system had been performing unnecessary cardiac procedures on healthy patients since at least 2002.

Doctors sent sick patients away and made them return as cardiology outpatients, so they could cash in on generous financial incentives, it is alleged. The fraudulent activity is alleged to have taken place for more than a year at the hospital which was only opened in 2013. But hospital officials are continuing to insist patient care was not compromised in the suspected scam. When cardiology patients were assessed, some were being told to return at a later date for their procedure, so they could be treated as outpatients. This would allow the doctor to bill Medicare for the appointment, topping up their salary which can already range from $200,000-$400,000-a-year.

Another cardiologist is said to have performed cardiac catheterizations on patients from at least January 2006 to February 2012 during which times he is alleged to have falsely recorded the existence or extent of coronary artery blockages in the patients' medical records. A coronary stent is not considered medically necessary unless a patient is diagnosed with a blockage of at least 70 percent. Investigators said that the doctor sought to increase his profit margin by performing the operations and then submitting false claims to Medicare, Medicaid and private insurance companies.

The cardiologist implanted potentially dangerous cardiac stents in the arteries of as many as 585 patients who didn't need them. He managed to perform 585 procedures in two years, from 2007 to 2009. Medicare paid $3.8 million of the $6.6 million charged for the treatments. The report reveals that the doctor was a favorite son of Abbott Laboratories, the company that manufactured the stents. Indeed, in August of 2008, Abbott celebrated the fact that the handy doctor had inserted 30 of the company's cardiac stents into trusting patients in a single day: "Two days later, an Abbott sales representative spent

$2,159 to buy a whole, slow-smoked pig, peach cobbler and other fixings for a barbecue dinner at the doctor's home."

The hospital encouraged the doctor to implant those tiny mesh tubes in his patients' arteries. Certainly, hospital executive knew that they were making handsome profits on the doctor's stent procedures. This is why they paid him those "bonuses" to shepherd unwitting patients to their Cath-lab where doctors can diagnose heart attacks, and quickly open arteries.

Health care consumers need to identify these health care fraudsters and report them to attempt to salvage the health care system. People need to remember that he/she could receive a monetary reward for being a whistle blower.

Whistle blowers are people who expose unethical or illegal wrongdoing within companies by reporting it internally to superiors or externally to the media, government authorities, or specialized attorneys. They can be either current or past employees (insiders), or outside individuals who are familiar with the unlawful conduct, and are not required to be U.S. citizens. If you properly report Medicare fraud, you may be entitled to a significant whistleblower reward.

29. Dermatology Fraud

Dermatology is the branch of medicine dealing with the skin, nails, hair and its diseases. It is a specialty with both medical and surgical aspects. A dermatologist treats diseases, in the widest sense, and some cosmetic problems with the skin, scalp, hair, and nails.

According to an indictment, a doctor intentionally misdiagnosed patients with skin cancer and performed unnecessary and invasive Mohs micrographic surgery on benign skin tissue. He then submitted claims to healthcare benefit programs using skin cancer diagnosis codes and fake certifications that these procedures had been medically necessary.

The indictment also states that the doctor billed insurers for Mohs surgeries that he never performed, and that he allegedly directed his staff to improperly dispose of medical waste at his offices. He is also charged with directing unlicensed and unqualified medical assistants to perform wound closures during follow-up visits, including complex suturing and skin grafts, on patients who underwent Mohs surgery. During these procedures, the doctor was allegedly with other patients at different office locations; so critical decisions about patient care were left up to the medical assistants. These procedures were "fraudulently" billed to health insurance companies as if the doctor had performed or personally supervised them.

A west suburban dermatologist has been accused of defrauding Medicare and private insurance companies for millions of dollars over several years, according to federal authorities. This doctor who runs a Center for Dermatology & Skin Cancer was indicted In U.S. District Court 3 on four counts of wire fraud and three counts of mail fraud. He is accused of submitting false claims for hundreds of patients,

The FBI alleges that the dermatologist falsely diagnosed patients with sun-induced skin lesions that can become cancerous and subsequently billed Medicare, Blue Cross Blue Shield of Illinois, Aetna and Humana for ineffective treatments. Between 2003 and 2010, the FBI alleges that the doctor also falsified patients' records to support medically unnecessary procedures, including the removal of more than 1,000 lesions from patients, o

Another dermatologist has been accused of intentionally misdiagnosing patients with skin cancer and performing unnecessary surgeries as part of a complex health-care fraud scheme. This dermatologist was indicted by a federal grand jury in on 60 counts of fraud, aggravated identity theft and other charges.

Another physician, a dermatologist, has agreed to pay $26.1 million to resolve allegations that he violated the False Claims Act by accepting illegal kickbacks from a pathology laboratory and by billing the Medicare program for medically unnecessary services, the Justice Department announced today. The settlement is the largest ever with an individual under the False Claims Act in the Middle District of Florida and one of the largest with an individual under the False Claims Act in U.S. history.

The government alleged that, in or around 1997, a dermatologist entered into an illegal kickback arrangement with a pathology laboratory, a clinical laboratory in Tampa, Fla., and a pathologist and the owner of a laboratory, in an effort to increase the lab's referral business. Under that agreement, the doctor allegedly sent biopsy specimens for Medicare beneficiaries to TPL for testing and diagnosis. In return, the laboratory allegedly provided the doctor a diagnosis on a pathology report that included a signature line for the doctor to make it appear to Medicare that he had performed the diagnostic work that the laboratory had performed.

The government alleged that the doctor then billed the Medicare program for the laboratory work, passing it off as his own, for which he received more than $6 million in Medicare payments. In addition, the government asserted that, in furtherance of his agreement with the laboratory; the doctor substantially increased the number of skin biopsies he performed on Medicare patients, thus increasing the referral business for the laboratory.

The government further alleged that, in addition to his involvement in the alleged kickback scheme, the doctor also performed thousands of unnecessary skin surgeries known as adjacent tissue transfers on Medicare beneficiaries. Adjacent tissue transfers are complicated, and often time-consuming procedures physicians sometimes use to close a defect resulting from the removal of a growth on a patient's skin.

A federal jury has convicted a Chicago dermatologist on fraud charges for billing health-insurance programs for purported precancerous treatments that were not medically necessary. Prosecutors say from 2007 to 2013, a doctor, of Chicago, submitted claims to multiple health-insurance programs, falsely claiming that his treatments were medically necessary to treat actinic keratosis, a pre-cancerous condition that he knew many of his patients did not actually have. The doctor documented the false claims by including in his patients' charts fictitious diagnoses of actinic keratosis that were not based on the patients' actual signs and symptoms.

The owners of an Atlanta-based medical practice have agreed to pay the federal government more than $3.2 million to settle Medicare fraud allegations, raising questions about how they funded their lavish lifestyle. The settlement came nearly two months after a news channel first reported on complaints of improper billing by a dermatologist, which is owned by a doctor and her husband. The couple lives in country singer Kenny Rogers' former mansion in Atlanta and owns two Rolls Royces, a Bentley and an Aston-Martin. According to the settlement agreement, the improper Medicare billing fueled Family Dermatology's rapid expansion to more than 40 practices in nine states by 2012. The message is medical providers need to comply with federal law.

The prosecution said the government found the doctors required physicians who worked for them to submit skin samples to a pathology laboratory the couple also owned, violating the Stark Statute. The couple then billed Medicare for those services.

But a former clinic medical assistant said the company's questionable practices weren't limited to Medicare. The medical assistant, who worked at the clinic in Pennsylvania in 2013 and 2014, said the office was inundated with complaints of double billing. We had health insurance companies calling us saying 'we paid this,'" said the employee. "It's embarrassing having to tell the patient, 'I have no explanation for you.' What kind of company does that look like? While the doctors were living luxuriously, these patients are paying for it." The medical assistant said she also saw the doctor regularly up code office visits on bills, which could bring in more money.

The doctor was always charging level three billing even though she was only spending two to five minutes in a room with a patient," said Kohler. Level three is supposed to be reserved for face-to-face visits which last 15 minutes. The doctors reported $36 million revenue in 2012, the company allegedly stopped paying many of its vendors and office landlords, forcing offices to close. Some physicians alleged they were owed hundreds of thousands of dollars after Family Dermatology stopped paying them.

A settlement has been reached in a federal investigation into allegations that a Jacksonville-based dermatology practice knowingly billed the government for services that were cosmetic and not medically necessary, according to the U.S. Attorney's Office.

A doctor, was convicted of 31 counts of fraud for overcharging insurance companies for procedures he did not perform. The doctor frequently removed growths (sometimes freckles or blemishes) after scaring patients into believing they were precancerous. He also double-billed for visits by falsely claiming that patients had impetigo, a highly contagious bacterial infection.

The judge found the fraud totaled more than $1 million. Prosecutors daubed the doctor as a doctor driven by greed, so arrogant that he continued to rip off insurance companies and hundreds of patients even after audits and warnings in the 1990s, after agents raided his office in 2001, and after he was criminally charged in August 2006. He also cut corners, reusing medical equipment without properly cleaning it, authorities said. Witnesses testified that he used braided, absorbable sutures, pulling them all the way through a patient's wound. He then reused leftovers on another patient, a "Third World" practice that could lead to infection, an expert said.

A doctor was indicted Tuesday on 60 counts of health care fraud, aggravated identity theft and obstruction of justice. The indictment spans three years, between 2009 and 2012. Among other allegations, the doctor was accused of intentionally misdiagnosing patients with skin cancer and performing unnecessary, expensive treatments. The doctor was also charged with allowing unqualified assistants to perform complicated procedures related to wound care and with directing staff to improperly dispose of medical waste. The indictment mentioned multiple instances of the doctor billing healthcare benefit programs for services which were not performed. It is also alleged he billed those programs for biopsy reports which he paid other professionals to prepare for him.

Another dermatologist allegedly pocketed tens of millions of dollars from Medicare by ordering medically unnecessary biopsies, falsely diagnosing patients with cancer, performing unnecessary radiation treatments on patients, and illegally billing those biopsies and radiation treatments. The judgment entered against this doctor, and his medical practice is $18,017,382.1.

A dermatologist was charged in a seven-count indictment returned with defrauding Medicare and private health insurance companies by submitting false claims for hundreds of patients resulting in millions of dollars of losses. This doctor falsely diagnosed patients with actinic keratosis, or sun-induced skin lesions that have the potential to become cancerous, and then billed Medicare, Blue Cross Blue Shield of Illinois, Aetna, and Humana for treatments that were ineffective and falsely documented.

He allegedly performed thousands of medically unnecessary skin surgeries on his patients in order to increase his overall revenue. The bulk of these surgeries, known as adjacent tissue transfers or "local flaps", were performed on Medicare patients. Dermatologists utilize adjacent skin transfers after removing certain skin defects, such as cancerous lesions or benign growths. It is a common procedure among patients age 60 and over, making it easily justifiable for this doctor to submit reimbursement claims to Medicare.

When performing an adjacent skin transfer, a physician surgically transplants a section of healthy skin onto a skin defect. This is done by simply cutting a flap from the healthy skin lying directly adjacent to the defect. The healthy tissue is then folded or "flapped" over the skin defect and sutured into place, forming a protective covering. According to the complaint, this doctor allegedly performed thousands of these unnecessary adjacent skin transfers and received around $6 million in Medicare reimbursements. Thanks, in part, to genetic tests that assess cancer risk. He said military insurance, called Tricare, and reimbursed the most for a single test. Tests were conducted and billed by a lab in Dallas, which offered another test a drug screening. And that screening made the lab more than $5 million dollars from Tricare last year.

Soldiers would line up every day in this parking lot by the dozens and provide their DNA, urine and Tricare ID cards in exchange for a $50 Wal-Mart gift card. They said they had this clinical research going, and that they paid you by Wal-Mart cards, so you'd give your urine," she said.

Documents show these doctors billed Tricare 418 separate times for unneeded screening for dozens of drugs like PCP, cocaine and methadone. This is nearly $7,000 at taxpayer's expense. And this wasn't the only place near Fort Hood where soldiers lined up. There was also a storefront a few blocks away. They were only there a little while before setting up shop at a more professional-looking site.

Investigators also alleged a dermatologist substantially increased the number of skin biopsies he performed on Medicare patients and performed thousands of unnecessary skin surgeries known as adjacent tissue transfers to obtain Medicare reimbursements for them, according to the statement.

The worrisome blotches that drove elderly patients to a dermatologist's offices in Okeechobee and Port St. Lucie could have been anything. However, whether they were warts, irritated skin or even freckles, the diagnosis from the dermatologist, who lives in a sprawling $28 million oceanfront mansion in Palm Beach, was typically the same: skin cancer.

The allegations, first made in a whistle blower lawsuit filed in U.S. District Court by a competing Palm Beach County dermatologist, were investigated by federal attorneys who used them to build a multi-million-dollar health-care fraud case against the doctor. According to the allegations, this doctor failed to follow basic regulations by allowing unlicensed, untrained, and unsupervised staff members to perform highly technical procedures. For example, the allegations reveal that the dermatologist routinely allowed unlicensed medical assistants to perform radiation therapy on patients often without adequate supervision. According to the whistle blowers'' assertions, the medical assistants lacked "basic knowledge" of how to perform radiation therapy and should not have been permitted to perform this type of procedure on patients without the proper training.

One doctor, working diligently filed his first complaint in December 2013. According to the complaint, the doctor in question required his physician assistants to perform up to 50 biopsies each day, and he instructed them to perform biopsies on skin disorders for which biopsies were not appropriate, such as acne, dried skin, warts, and freckles. Once the biopsies were completed, the doctor being investigated sent the specimens to Dr. another individual, a physician who operates a laboratory in Coral Gables, FL. The suit alleged that both doctors were involved in an illegal kickback scheme in which one doctor allowed the other doctor to bill Medicare for the work performed as if it were performed by the other doctor, and in exchange the first doctor received remuneration.

The complaint further alleged that the doctor in question falsely diagnosed benign skin conditions as cancerous, affording the opportunity to recommend that such patients undergo radiation therapy, which generated extra billing opportunities. In addition to defrauding the government, this practice presented a considerable risk to patients, as radiation therapy presents an increased risk of cancer, and can also be harmful to healthy skin.

In another case, a noted dermatologist pleaded not guilty to writing bogus prescriptions for her own benefit. The doctor was arrested earlier in the day at her Park Avenue office. She is charged with criminal possession of narcotics and fraud. The doctor is accused of writing fraudulent prescriptions using former and current patients' names without their knowledge. The celebrity skin doctor would allegedly tell pharmacists she was filling the prescriptions for patients, but instead took them herself.

Health care consumers need to identify these health care fraudsters and report them to attempt to salvage the health care system. People need to remember that he/she could receive a monetary reward for being a whistle blower.

Whistle blowers are people who expose unethical or illegal wrongdoing within companies by reporting it internally to superiors or externally to the media, government authorities, or specialized attorneys. They can be either current or past employees (insiders), or outside individuals who are familiar with the unlawful conduct, and are not required to be U.S. citizens. If you properly report Medicare fraud, you may be entitled to a significant whistleblower reward.

30. Emergency Medicine Fraud

Emergency medicine, formerly known in some countries as accident and emergency medicine, is the medical specialty involving care for undifferentiated and unscheduled patients with illnesses or injuries requiring immediate medical attention. In their role as first-line providers, emergency physicians are responsible for initiating investigations and interventions to diagnose and/or treat patients in the acute phase (including initial resuscitation and stabilization), coordinating care with physicians from other specialties, and making decisions regarding a patient's need for hospital admission, observation, or discharge.

If you were an uninsured patient billed an excessive amount for emergency-room treatment at a major hospital, you may be the victim of emergency-room overcharges. An emergency-room bill for uninsured patients is often much greater than the emergency-room cost or ER bill that is submitted to an insurance company for the same ER treatment.

A doctor in Kingston, Ontario, was sentenced to 30 months in the penitentiary after defrauding the Ontario Health Insurance Plan of almost $600,000.Columbia HCA admitted to submitting a long list of charges, including submitting inflated bills and expenses to the government, exaggerating the seriousness of diagnoses to increase Medicare reimbursement, and providing doctors with kickbacks for patient referrals. HCA agreed to pay more than $840 million in criminal fines, penalties, and damages for unlawful billing practices.

Emergency physicians tend not to be involved in self-referrals, although it is possible that EPs may have partial ownership in Holter monitor services, clinical laboratory services, or radiology centers. There certainly has been the historical precedent for primary care physicians to build up a private practice by referring patients to themselves while moonlighting in the ED. It is unclear how the Ethics in Patient Referral Act (the so-called Stark I and II Acts) will affect this practice.

Judging by their bills, it would appear that elderly patients treated in the emergency room at Baylor Medical Center in Irving, Texas, are among the sickest in the country, far sicker than patients at most other hospitals. In 2008, the hospital billed Medicare for the two most expensive levels of care for eight of every 10 patients it treated and released from its emergency-room, almost twice the national average, according to a Center for Public Integrity analysis. Among those claims, 64 percent of the total were for the most expensive level of care. But the charges may have more to do with billing practices than sicker patients. A Baylor representative conceded hospital billing for emergency-room care "did not align with industry trends," but said that the hospital since 2009 has reined in its charges.

The Texas hospital's billing pattern is far from unique. Between 2001 and 2008, hospitals across the country dramatically increased their Medicare billing for emergency-room care, adding more than $1 billion to the cost of the program to taxpayers, a Center investigation has found. The fees are based upon a system of billing codes so-called evaluation and management codes that makes higher payments for treatments that require more time and resources.

Use of the top two most expensive codes for emergency-room care nationwide nearly doubled, from 25 percent to 45 percent of all claims, during the time period examined. In many cases, these claims were not for treating patients with life-threatening injuries. Instead, the claims the Center analyzed included only patients who were sent home from the emergency room without being admitted to the hospital. Often, they were treated for seemingly minor injuries and complaints.

While taxpayers footed most of the bill, the charges also hit elderly patients in the pocketbook, increasing the amount of their 20-percent co-payments for emergency-room care. Hospitals and federal officials say the rise has likely been caused by an increase in sicker patients seeking care in emergency rooms, more accurate billing on the part of hospitals, and an increasing number of options for patients who aren't as sick options that include retail-based clinics and urgent care facilities. The Center's investigation found that the surge in billing also reflects lax government oversight, confusion about proper billing standards, and widespread payment errors that have plagued Medicare for more than a decade. And the data suggest that some hospitals are working the billing system and its flaws to maximize payments.

Hospital industry insiders say it's no secret that hospitals are pushing the limits to bill higher-priced Medicare codes, a practice known as up coding. Few hospitals, however, are being scrutinized. Medicare officials are aware of the rising expense of emergency-room billing for evaluation and management services, but the agency has downplayed the problem and done little to verify the accuracy of hospital emergency room charges. Instead, it has given hospitals a free hand to set their own billing policies, with little agency guidance and even less auditing.

Medicare lacks rules for hospital ER billing. Since 2000, hospitals have chosen among five codes to bill Medicare and other insurers for evaluating emergency-room patients and coordinating their treatment. This hospital "facility fee," which can add millions of dollars to the hospital's bottom line in the course of a year, ranges from $50 to $324, depending on which code is chosen for any given case. It comes on top of physician charges.

The system dates back to a change in federal law requiring hospitals be paid a set fee for services, rather than a blanket payment based upon the cost of providing care, which was meant to save the program money. Yet instead of developing specialized billing codes just for hospitals, CMS since 2000 has required hospitals to file claims using a set of codes developed and licensed for physician billing by the American Medical Association so-called Current Procedural Terminology, or CPT, codes. The lack of specific hospital codes, or guidelines for how hospitals should use physician codes, has left the system open to broad interpretation by hospitals.

The United States District Court for the Western District of North Carolina, in response to a Department of Justice motion, has unsealed a whistle blower lawsuit filed against Health Management Associates, Inc., ("HMA") and Emergency Medical Services Corporation ("EMCARE") alleging that they cheated the Medicare and Medicaid Programs in its hospitals across the United States by: Admitting emergency-room patients to HMA hospitals when it was not necessary, paying kickbacks to emergency rooms to incentive and pay them to order expensive emergency-room services and admit patients when it was not essential and to order costly diagnostic tests that are unnecessary.

In one of at least eight whistle blower lawsuits against hospital chain Health Management Associates, two emergency-room physicians allege the company offered kickbacks in exchange for admitting patients and submitted false claims to Medicare and Medicaid programs for unnecessary admissions and medical procedures. HMA is accused of telling emergency-room physicians that 75 percent of all Medicare patients should be admitted.

Drug Task Force agents confirmed Friday an emergency medicine doctor with Union General Hospital was arrested in Fannin County earlier this week. The doctor was booked into jail for writing prescriptions for himself and attempting to have them filled. Agents were investigating another case at Walmart in Blue Ridge that morning and Walmart had given them information that the doctor had attempted to pass two prescriptions there, earlier that day and those prescriptions were denied. The doctor is an emergency medicine physician.

Another lawsuit alleges HMA provided illegal remuneration to a physician practice group in North Port for referring and admitting patients to Charlotte Regional, cheating the federal government out of $100 million to $150 million. Echoing other complaints across the country, two Charlotte-area emergency room doctors allege the for-profit company that owns hospitals in Mooresville and Statesville offered them illegal kickbacks to order unnecessary tests and admit more patients to increase corporate revenues.

An employee of a small Nevada hospital where she worked suspected that the hospital was overcharging Medicare and other health insurers for some emergency room services. She ran Boulder City Hospital's health information department, which helped apply the complex series of Medicare billing codes doctors and hospitals must use to get paid for treating the sick. But she alleged in a lawsuit that her bosses told her to "back off" when she doubted the accuracy of the coding and fired her in May when she refused to sign off on it

It's no secret that hospital bills in the U.S., especially ones from the E.R. can often hit astronomical proportions. According to a recent cost study conducted by researchers at Stanford University, the University of Minnesota, the University of California, San Francisco and the Ecologic Institute, the median charge for an emergency-room journey in the U.S. comes in at $1,233. But where it really gets interesting is when you look at the specific reasons for those E.R. visits: The researchers found that the treatment price for a headache could range from $15 to a whopping $17,797. As for a sprained ankle, it could set someone back a paltry $4 or up to $24,110!

Most emergency-room prices are inflated based upon the rates at which insurance companies will reimburse the hospital on a patient's behalf. That's why a single aspirin can cost $30 per pill in the E.R., which is more than six times the price for a bottle of them at the drug store. On the flip side, patients will often contact the hospital or surgeon's billing office to ask for a cost reduction, further adding to the inconsistency in pricing. It's a practice that often works in a patient's favor, says billing advocacy specialist Sharon Salters of Medical Cost Advocate, a professional medical bill negotiation service.

Much of the ongoing health care reform debate has focused on unnecessary health care expenses, specifically, medical bills that rack up without demonstrably improving peoples' health. According to Peter Orszag, the director of the federal Office of Management and Budget, about $700 billion, or 5 percent of the U.S. gross domestic product, is wasted on unnecessary care, such as extra costs related to medical errors, defensive medicine, and just plain fraud.

At the center of this discussion are "unnecessary" ER visits for minor conditions colds, headaches, and feverish babies that could be handled more cheaply in doctors' offices. If we could only convince patients to take their stubbed toes to urgent-care clinics or primary-care offices instead of ERs, the thinking goes, we could save a significant amount of money and help fix the whole health care debacle.

Judging by their bills, it would appear that elderly patients treated in the emergency room at Baylor Medical Center in Irving, Texas, are among the sickest in the country far sicker than patients at most other hospitals. In 2008, the hospital billed Medicare for the two most expensive levels of care for eight of every 10 patients it treated and released from its emergency room almost twice the national average, according to a Center for Public Integrity analysis. Among those claims, 64 percent of the total was for the most expensive level of care.

But the charges may have more to do with billing practices than sicker patients. A Baylor representative conceded hospital billing for emergency-room care "did not align with industry trends," but said that the hospital since 2009 has reined in its charges.

The Texas hospital's billing pattern is far from unique. Between 2001 and 2008, hospitals across the country dramatically increased their Medicare billing for emergency-room care, adding more than $1 billion to the cost of the program to taxpayers, a Center investigation has found. The fees are based upon a system of billing codes so-called evaluation and management codes that makes higher payments for treatments that require more time and resources.

Use of the top two most expensive codes for emergency-room care nationwide nearly doubled, from 25 percent to 45 percent of all claims, during the time period examined. In many cases, these claims were not for treating patients with life-threatening injuries. Instead, the claims the Center analyzed included only patients who were sent home from the emergency room without being admitted to the hospital. Often, they were treated for seemingly minor injuries and complaints.

Between August 2011 and September 7, 2011, a doctor was employed as an emergency-room physician at a Hospital. During that time, he devised a scheme whereby on September 7, 2011, his girlfriend reported to the emergency room at the Hospital and pretended to suffer from a medical condition known as trigeminal neuralgia. The defendant then performed an apparent examination of her, fraudulently diagnosed her as suffering from trigeminal neuralgia and issued a prescription to her for Dilauded, a controlled substance.

In reality, the girlfriend was not suffering from this condition and had no medical need for the drug Dilaudid. In participating in this illegal scheme, the defendant defrauded the Hospital and also aided and abetted his girlfriend in obtaining a controlled substance by fraud.

A whistle blower case alleging that Florida Hospital and six affiliates knowingly over billed Medicare "tens of millions of dollars" in radiology services has widened to include the hospitals' emergency departments, according to an amended complaint filed this month. The new complaint against Adventist Health System, which owns the hospitals, alleges that routine billing fraud occurred in the emergency departments from 2001 to 2008 and possibly longer.

Most insurers, including Medicare, reimburse at higher rates for inpatient procedures than they do for outpatient versions of the same treatment. According to one lawsuit doctors at Health Management were under particularly intense pressure to milk more money out of retirement-age people: They had a mandate to make sure that half of all patients over age 65 who visited the emergency room got admitted into the hospital, and doctors' progress towards that goal was tracked.

A First Choice emergency medical center appeared last year where a Blockbuster Video outlet once stood, near a strip center. The glossy new facility has the latest equipment, from a CT scanner to a portable X-ray. An in-house lab provides quick test results. There are free snacks and a Keurig coffee machine, and a well-appointed children's examining room that has an original undersea wall mural and cartoons on the TV.

By locating in well-trafficked, convenient and often affluent areas where potential customers already shop, such as free standing medical centers provide an easy alternative to the hospital ERs with their long waits and sometimes gritty settings. Nationally, they've doubled to more than 400 since 2009, according to Kaiser Health Care News. However, there is a growing backlash to the lucrative medical facilities, where sprained ankles, stitches and other simple procedures can cost upward of $1,000. And health insurer Aetna is suing two ER centers in Texas, alleging fraud.

Like hospital ERs, the doctor- and investor-owned centers benefit from emergency-room cases that could have been treated far more cheaply at a doctor's office or urgent care facility. Such cases represent 27.1 percent of ER cases, according to a 2010 study by the National Institutes of Health. If those cases were treated at the cheaper clinics, $4.4 billion could be saved annually, the study estimated.

There's enough profit in the expanding market segment to snare the interest of private-equity investors and large hospital groups, which don't want to lose market share. Baylor Healthcare System and Texas Health Resources have both entered the competition in North Texas. Baylor is partnering with for-profit Emerus Emergency Facilities to set up downsized hospitals with inpatient beds while and Texas Health Harris Methodist has developed a center with both ER and primary care units.

When First Choice's parent corporation, Adeptus Health, became a publicly traded stock in June, mandated disclosures offered a glimpse into the industry. Last year, First Choice, the nation's biggest free standing ER chain, collected an average $1,500 per patient and treated 77,044, according to the prospectus filed with the Securities and Exchange Commission.

Blue Cross has issued literature explaining the differences. "Free standing ERs often look a lot like urgent care centers, but costs are higher, just as if you go to the ER at a hospital," the quick reference guide cautions. It also offers a smart phone app for finding the nearest urgent-care clinic and staffs a 24-hour nurse line to rein in higher costs at free standing ER centers.

It has been found that the free-standing ERs don't really treat emergencies. In fact, for real emergencies they call 911 or get an ambulance for the patient to be transferred to an actual hospital ER. The arrangements between the free-standing ER and hospital are usually a sham with the only real interaction between the entities is a split of the facility fee that can now be charged.

Health care consumers need to identify these health care fraudsters and report them to attempt to salvage the health care system. People need to remember that he/she could receive a monetary reward for being a whistle blower.

Whistle blowers are people who expose unethical or illegal wrongdoing within companies by reporting it internally to superiors or externally to the media, government authorities, or specialized attorneys. They can be either current or past employees (insiders), or outside individuals who are familiar with the unlawful conduct, and are not required to be U.S. citizens. If you properly report Medicare fraud, you may be entitled to a significant whistleblower reward.

31. Endocrinology Fraud

Endocrinology is a branch of biology and medicine dealing with the endocrine system, its diseases, and its specific secretions known as hormones. There are not any significant endocrinology fraud cases reported at the time of the writing of this book.

A doctor has been charged in federal court in Manhattan with a two-year-long conspiracy to illegally distribute the painkiller oxycodone from a clinic in Boston, Massachusetts. This doctor sold prescriptions for more than 1,000 medically unnecessary oxycodone pills, charging hundreds or thousands of dollars for cursory or nonexistent medical exams, according to a criminal complaint.

An endocrinologist was fingered by an informant who secretly taped the doctor urging him to bring a list of names to use on phony prescriptions, and on another occasion taking $5,000, the complaint said. The confidential source told the FBI that he had begun buying prescriptions written for him and another man whom the doctor never met, the complaint said.

With respect to the field of endocrinology, there are only a few cases of fraud that involve billing for office visits that were never done.

Health care consumers need to identify these health care fraudsters and report them to attempt to salvage the health care system. People need to remember that he/she could receive a monetary reward for being a whistle blower.

Whistle blowers are people who expose unethical or illegal wrongdoing within companies by reporting it internally to superiors or externally to the media, government authorities, or specialized attorneys. They can be either current or past employees (insiders), or outside individuals who are familiar with the unlawful conduct, and are not required to be U.S. citizens. If you properly report Medicare fraud, you may be entitled to a significant whistleblower reward.

32. Family Practice Fraud

A primary-care physician is a physician who provides both the first contact for a person with an undiagnosed health concern as well as continuing care of varied medical conditions, not limited by cause, organ system, or diagnosis. Since recently, the term has been primarily used in the United States. In the past in the US and still in the United Kingdom (and in many other English-speaking countries), the equivalent term was/is a general practitioner.

Family medicine (FM), formerly family practice (FP), is a specialty devoted to comprehensive health care for people of all ages; the specialist is named a family physician or family doctor. Family medicine (FM), formerly family practice (FP), is a specialty devoted to comprehensive health care for people of all ages; the specialist is named a family physician or family doctor.

All physicians first complete medical school (MD, MBBS, or DO). To become primary care physicians, medical school graduates then undertake postgraduate training in primary care programs, such as family medicine pediatrics or internal medicine. Primary care is the day-to-day healthcare given by a health care provider. Typically, this provider acts as the first contact and principal point of continuing care for patients within a healthcare system, and coordinates other specialist care that the patient may need. Depending on the nature of the health condition, patients may then be referred for secondary or tertiary care.

A Manhattan, N.Y.-based physician and eight others have been charged for allegedly distributing oxycodone pills through a Manhattan-based drug ring, according to a news release by the Drug Enforcement Administration. A family physician allegedly wrote oxycodone prescriptions to patients without a legitimate need for the medication between Sept. 2009 and Aug. 2010. Co-conspirators helped the individuals fill the prescriptions and arranged to resell the oxycodone to third parties. Two others, allegedly obtained oxycodone prescriptions despite having no medical need for the medication, then used their government-provided health benefits to fill their prescriptions and sold the pills to others.

Approximately 11,000 oxycodone pills were obtained and distributed by members of the drug ring. According to the New York

State Office of the Medicaid Inspector General, over the course of the conspiracy $997,128 of $4,392,832 in Medicaid drug expenses for medications prescribed by the doctor was attributable to OxyContin prescriptions.

The five most important Federal fraud and abuse laws that apply to physicians are the False Claims Act (FCA), the Anti-Kickback Statute (AKS), the Physician Self-Referral Law (Stark law), the Exclusion Authorities, and the Civil Monetary Penalties Law (CMPL). Government agencies, including the Department of Justice, the Department of Health & Human Services Office of Inspector General (OIG), and the Centers for Medicare & Medicaid Services (CMS), are charged with enforcing these laws. It is crucial for a primary-care physician to understand these laws not only because following them is the right thing to do, but also because violating them could result in criminal penalties, civil fines, exclusion from the Federal health care programs, or loss of one's medical license from the State medical board.

The civil FCA protects the Government from being overcharged or sold shoddy goods or services. It is illegal to submit claims for payment to Medicare or Medicaid that you know or should know are false or fraudulent. Filing false claims may result in fines of up to three times the programs' loss plus $11,000 per claim filed. Under the civil FCA, each instance of an item or a service billed to Medicare or Medicaid counts as a claim, so fines can add up quickly. The fact that a claim results from a kickback or is made in violation of the Stark law also may render it false or fraudulent, creating liability under the civil FCA as well as the AKS or Stark law.

Under the civil FCA, no specific intent to defraud is required. The civil FCA defines "knowing" to include not only actual knowledge but also instances in which the person acted in deliberate ignorance or reckless disregard of the truth or falsity of the information. Further, the civil FCA contains a whistle blower provision that allows a private individual to file a lawsuit on behalf of the United States and entitles that whistle blower to a percentage of any recoveries. Whistle blowers could be current or ex-business partners, hospital or office staff, patients, or competitors.

There also is a criminal FCA (18 U.S.C. § 287). Criminal penalties for submitting false claims include imprisonment and criminal fines. Physicians have gone to prison for submitting false health care claims. OIG also may impose administrative civil monetary penalties for false or fraudulent claims, as discussed below.

Anti-Kickback Statute is a criminal law that prohibits the knowing and willful payment of "remuneration" to induce or reward patient referrals or the generation of business involving any item or service payable by the Federal health care programs (e.g., drugs, supplies, or health care services for Medicare or Medicaid patients). Remuneration includes anything of value and can take many forms besides cash, such as free rent, expensive hotel stays and meals, and excessive compensation for medical directorships or consultancies. In some industries, it is acceptable to reward those who refer business to you. However, in the Federal health care programs, paying for referrals is a crime. The statute covers the payers of kickbacks-those who offer or pay remuneration- as well as the recipients of kickbacks-those who solicit or receive remuneration. Each party's intent is a key element of their liability under the AKS.

Criminal penalties and administrative sanctions for violating the Anti-Kickback Statute (AKS) include fines, jail terms, and exclusion from participation in the Federal health care programs. Under the CMPL, physicians who pay or accept kickbacks also face penalties of up to $50,000 per kickback plus three times the amount of the remuneration.

As a physician, one is an attractive target for kickback schemes because a primary-care physician can be a source of referrals for fellow physicians or other health care providers and suppliers. A primary-care physician decides what drugs patients' use, which specialists they see, and what health care services and supplies they receive. The Physician Self-Referral Law, commonly referred to as the Stark law, prohibits physicians from referring patients to receive "designated health services" payable by Medicare or Medicaid from entities with which the physician or an immediate family member has a financial relationship, unless an exception applies. Financial relationships include both ownership/investment interests and compensation arrangements. For example, if a physician invests in an imaging center, the Stark law requires the resulting financial relationship to fit within an exception, or you may not refer patients to the facility, and the entity may not bill for the referred imaging services.

Allergy testing and immunotherapy schemes continue to pop up in primary care practices across the country, exposing patients and families to substandard diagnosis and treatment as well as raising the potential for fraudulent billing. However, there are deceptions too and here is how to recognize the signs of fraud. Primary care offices enter into agreements with third-party companies whereby a "certified allergy specialist" tests patients and recommends treatment. Patients are shuffled in for environmental and/or food allergy testing, and then offered immunotherapy, which may include either allergy shots or sublingual immunotherapy (SLIT) in which drops of the allergen are placed on the tongue. Many patients are unaware that SLIT is not currently approved and, therefore, not typically reimbursable by insurance.

Meanwhile, patients are unaware that these "certified allergy specialists" are not formally trained allergists. Many treatments recommended are inconsistent with established standards of practice designed to protect you as the patient. However, many primary care practices, some unknowingly, bill insurance companies. This is just one example of insurance billing fraud. Others include maximizing the number of allergens tested in order to maximize reimbursement; giving extremely low doses to avoid reactions, although reimbursement remains the same; and treating with a universal stock mix that contains many allergens a patient is not allergic to."

Many of these "certified allergy specialists" have no previous medical experience whatsoever and are given quotas for the number of patients they must test and put on allergy shots or risk losing their job. The researchers called it "low-value care." But, really, it was no-value care. They studied how often people received one of twenty-six tests or treatments that scientific and professional organizations have consistently determined to have no benefit or to be outright harmful.

Their list included doing an EEG for an uncomplicated headache (EEGs are for diagnosing seizure disorders, not headaches), or doing a CT or MRI scan for low-back pain in patients without any signs of a neurological problem (studies consistently show that scanning such patients adds nothing except cost), or putting a coronary-artery stent in patients with stable cardiac disease (the likelihood of a heart attack or death after five years is unaffected by the stent). In just a single year, the researchers reported, twenty-five to forty-two per cent of Medicare patients received at least one of the twenty-six useless tests and treatments.

Virtually every family in the country, the research indicates, has been subject to over testing and over treatment in one form or another. The costs appear to take thousands of dollars out of the paychecks of every household each year. Researchers have come to refer to financial as well as physical "toxicities" of inappropriate care—including reduced spending on food, clothing, education, and shelter. Millions of people are receiving drugs that aren't helping them, operations that aren't going to make them better, and scans and tests that do nothing beneficial for them, and often cause harm.

If you have crushing chest pain and shortness of breath, you start with a high likelihood of having a serious heart condition, and an electrocardiogram has significant value. A heart tracing that doesn't look quite right usually means trouble. But, if you have no signs or symptoms of heart trouble, an electrocardiogram adds no useful information; a heart tracing that doesn't look quite right is mostly noise. Experts recommend against doing electrocardiograms on healthy people, but millions are done each year, anyway.

In another scam indictment alleged that from 2007 to 2010, two physicians falsely billed Medicare and Medicaid under vestibular diagnostic codes. They allegedly billed Medicare and Medicaid approximately $850,000 and were paid approximately $390,000. Vestibular problems are traditionally inner ear problems with the patients reporting chronic dizziness and balance problems. One of these physicians operated a family practice clinic in Houston while the other physician operated a rehabilitation center. According to the indictment, the family physician would send unlicensed persons into Medicare beneficiaries' homes to perform some types of vestibular testing. The family physician allegedly would then submit "super bills"" to the second individual and his billing contractor for this testing.

The indictment indicates that patients reported either that none of the testing was performed or that some form of testing was performed but not in the quantity that was actually billed. One patient's Medicare number was allegedly billed for more than 800 tests on 161 different days over the course of one year. Others were billed for more than 500 tests over a period of one year, according to the indictment. The patients, their families or their treating doctors reported that these patients did not need vestibular testing and did not complain of dizziness. The second individual allegedly billed Medicare and Medicaid for these diagnostic tests and split the paid claims with the family physician. The indictment indicates that the testing individual kept 35 percent, while the family physician received the remainder.

Medicare spending on doctors who make house calls rose to $236 million in 2012 a 40% increase since 2006. But the effort to help aging patients with limited mobility get medical care has been riddled with fraud due to lax regulations in some areas of the U.S. In Michigan, a fifth of all the spending on Medicare home visits nationwide takes place. In 2012, physicians in Michigan received Medicare funds for home visits equal to 42 other states combined. The result: family practice physician, and her husband, purported to specialize in providing injection and infusion therapies, have been convicted for their roles in a $2.3 million Medicare fraud scheme, according to a Department of Justice news release. According to prosecutors, these individuals falsified medical files to make it appear that the clinic's patients actually needed the medications being billed to Medicare. Between approximately Nov. 2006 and March 2007, the defendants submitted approximately $2.3 million in claims to Medicare for injection therapy services that were never provided and were not medically necessary. Medicare paid approximately $1.7 million of those claims.

A 67-year-old physician was arraigned Tuesday on multiple felony charges for a scheme in which he allegedly prescribed medication in exchange for money and sexual favors, an Attorney General announced. Another doctor was charged with two counts of first-degree criminal sexual conduct, one count of conducting a criminal enterprise-racketeering, one count of conspiracy to deliver controlled substances less than 50 grams and nine counts of Medicaid fraud-false claim. This doctor practiced as a doctor of osteopathic medicine at his family practice clinic.

Health care consumers need to identify these health care fraudsters and report them to attempt to salvage the health care system. People need to remember that he/she could receive a monetary reward for being a whistle blower.

Whistle blowers are people who expose unethical or illegal wrongdoing within companies by reporting it internally to superiors or externally to the media, government authorities, or specialized attorneys. They can be either current or past employees (insiders), or outside individuals who are familiar with the unlawful conduct, and are

not required to be U.S. citizens. If you properly report Medicare fraud, you may be entitled to a significant whistleblower reward.

33. Gastroenterology Fraud

According to the American College of Gastroenterology, Gastroenterology is the study of the normal function and diseases of the esophagus, stomach, small intestine, colon and rectum, pancreas, gallbladder, bile ducts and liver. A gastroenterologist needs to have a detailed understanding of the normal physiology of all the above-mentioned organs as well as motility through the intestines and gastrointestinal tract in order to maintain a healthy digestion, absorption of nutrients, removal of waste and metabolic processes. A gastroenterologist also needs to have a clear understanding of ailments affecting the organs of the gastrointestinal system.

Gastroenterologists deal with gastrointestinal tract ailments so tests that are performed in gastroenterology departments are usually tested to find out what's wrong with your stomach or intestines. EGD or esophagogastroduodenoscopy is a test where a fiberoptic camera is passed into the mouth, through the esophagus and into the stomach and sometimes into the duodenum (part of the small intestine) to find out if there are ulcers, bleeding, or benign/malignant tumors in your esophagus, stomach or duodenum.

Until recently, there was no way to find out if bleeding is occurring in a person's small intestines but a test called small bowel endoscopy changed all that. In this test, a person swallows a pill, which is a little bit larger than a normal-sized pill, which passes through the gastrointestinal tract. The capsule contains a small camera that transmits pictures of the inside of the small intestines to a receiver worn outside the body. The receiver usually looks like a girdle or a professional wrestling belt that is wrapped around the abdomen. The capsule will go through its normal tract, like food does, and is excreted via the rectum when a person defecates. The most common test performed in the department is colonoscopy. Colonoscopy is similar to EGD but the fiberoptic camera is passed through the rectum, and the colon (large intestine) is visualized through the camera.

According to court documents, a physician licensed in the State of Florida, who specializes in the field of gastroenterology, filed fraudulent income tax returns. The doctor's primary place of business was in Palm Beach, Florida. For the tax years 2004 to 2008, this doctor knowingly and willfully underreported his income from the above-mentioned entities. He received income in the form of direct compensation, distributions, and corporate funds and used these payments to cover personal expenditures. This resulted in the filing of false corporate and personal tax returns by the doctor.

He utilized funds from the company to pay for expenses related to a new home that he built in Manalapan, Florida, payments on condominiums that he had purchased, interior-design improvements to his residences, and tuition payments for his children. Some of these payments were then fraudulently classified as professional consulting, building repairs, and miscellaneous expenses by the referenced companies.

These falsified profit and loss statements, which included the improper payments, were used by a tax preparer to file his corporate and personal income tax returns. In fact, the AMA estimates that a basic colonoscopy takes 75 minutes of a physician's time. This includes the work performed before, during and after the scoping.

It doesn't take doctors this long to perform colonoscopies. In a magazine article, one Florida gastroenterologist said he routinely performs 16 procedures a day. This includes 12 colonoscopies. He said it generally takes him nine to 10 hours to complete this work in a day. However, according to the AMA estimates, that it should take that doctor 26 hours to perform all these procedures. So, either the doctor works more than twice as fast as the AMA says he should or he's being overpaid. The doctor is probably pushing to complete as many colon screenings as he can in one day to beef up his "bottom" line. And I'm sure he's not the only one. In fact, most gastroenterologists allot just 30 minutes for a routine colonoscopy. Without a doubt, the AMA is still way off base in its time estimate.

As a result, the taxpayers (through Medicare/Medicaid) foot the bill for three days of work. However, it only takes the doctor one day to do the work. The insurance companies overpay too because they use the same AMA estimates. However, from a health standpoint, there's an even bigger issue. As I mentioned earlier, some experts say colonoscopies aren't even the best screening tool for colorectal cancer.

From January 2006 to December 2007, a gastroenterology group occupied a suite owned by a hospital without paying any rent to the hospital, the release states. There was no written lease. In January 2008, the hospital and office entered into a written lease, but the hospital still failed to collect any monthly rent until August 2009, the government states. Between January 2006 and August 2009, the office was regularly referring Medicare patients to this hospital, and the hospital was submitting claims to Medicare for those patients, the release states.

The Stark Law prohibits physicians from referring patients to a hospital with whom they have an improper financial arrangement. Rental arrangements are improper when they lack a written lease or when their costs are not consistent with fair market values. The law is meant to ensure that a physician's medical judgment is based solely on the best interests of the patient and is not compromised by improper financial incentives.

A gastroenterologist, who was awarded four patents for drugs used to treat the liver disease Hepatitis C, was convicted last year in a scheme that bilked millions from insurance companies. The celebration is significant, as Las Vegas Endoscopy is the first independent endoscopy center to open in Clark County since 2008, when Las Vegas made national news for a horrifying scandal.

In February of that year, the Southern Nevada Health District informed 40,000 patients of an endoscopy Center of Southern Nevada that they had been exposed to Hepatitis C and HIV through unsafe practices at the center. An investigation in cooperation with the Centers for Disease Control and Prevention discovered unhygienic practices, including re-using syringes and single-use medications. The endoscopy Center and five sister clinics were shuttered. The gastroenterologist at the root of the outbreak was later found guilty of more than two dozen criminal counts, including second-degree murder, conspiracy and health care fraud, sentenced to life in state prison and 71 months in federal prison.

The doctors participated in a $96 million billing scheme that recruited 2,000 healthy people from all over the country to receive unnecessary surgeries in exchange for money or low cost surgery. The recruitment of patients, or "capping," is illegal in most states. Insurance companies paid the physician group more than $17 million during a 10-month period.

Recruiters, targeted employees from businesses in more than 32 states and covered by PPO insurance plans, as pre-approval from the insurance company would not be a requirement for surgery. More than 1,600 employers were affected by employees who were involved in this scheme. The cappers arranged transportation for the patients, scheduled the procedures, and coached the healthy patients on what to say. In exchange for undergoing surgery, the "patients" would receive a cash payment, usually between $300 and $1,000 per surgery, or credit toward free or discounted cosmetic procedures.

The doctors charged in this case are accused of participating in medical insurance fraud for performing medical procedures on healthy people with the knowledge that the patients were being recruited. These doctors are accused of performing 1,037 procedures, resulting in insurance billings for the facilities' fees alone that exceeded $30 million. Unity received more than $5.1 million in payment as a result of the surgeries performed by the doctors.

Many of the surgeries were performed on Saturdays and Sundays by the doctors. Often, they operated on members of the same household on the same day. The doctors are accused of ignoring basic medical protocols such as: 1) patients receiving surgeries on consecutive days instead of while under anesthesia; 2) doctors not meeting the patients prior to operating; 3) doctors not following up with patients after the procedure was completed; and 4) doctors not obtaining necessary medical information.

Colonic irrigation, which also can be expensive, has a considerable potential for harm. The process can be very uncomfortable, since the presence of the tube can induce severe cramps and pain. If the equipment is not adequately sterilized between treatments, disease germs from one person's large intestine can be transmitted to others. Several outbreaks of serious infections have been reported, including one in which contaminated equipment caused amebiasis in 36 people, 6 of whom died following bowel perforation. Cases of heart failure (from excessive fluid absorption into the bloodstream) and electrolyte imbalance have also been reported . Direct rectal perforation has also been reported .

No license or training is required to operate a colonic-irrigation device. In 1985, a California judge ruled that colonic irrigation is an invasive medical procedure that may not be performed by chiropractors and the California Health Department's Infectious Disease Branch stated: "The practice of colonic irrigation by chiropractors, physical therapists, or physicians should cease. Colonic irrigation can do no good, only harm." The National Council Against Health Fraud agrees.

In 2009, Dr. Edzard Ernst tabulated the therapeutic claims he found on the Web sites of six "professional organizations of colonic irrigations." The themes he found included detoxification, normalization of intestinal function, treatment of inflammatory bowel disease, and weight loss. He also found claims related to asthma, menstrual irregularities, circulatory disorders, skin problems, and improvements in energy levels. Searching Medline and Embase, he was unable to find a single controlled clinical trial that substantiated any of these claims.

Health care consumers need to identify these health care fraudsters and report them to attempt to salvage the health care system. People need to remember that he/she could receive a monetary reward for being a whistle blower.

Whistle blowers are people who expose unethical or illegal wrongdoing within companies by reporting it internally to superiors or externally to the media, government authorities, or specialized attorneys. They can be either current or past employees (insiders), or outside individuals who are familiar with the unlawful conduct, and are not required to be U.S. citizens. If you properly report Medicare fraud, you may be entitled to a significant whistleblower reward.

34. Geriatrics Fraud

A geriatrician is a doctor who specializes in care for people 65 and older. Just as a pediatrician tends to the needs of a child, a geriatrician cares for the special needs of changing seniors. Geriatricians approach each patient's needs individually, and possess the knowledge and expertise needed to accommodate seniors. They are typically board-certified in internal medicine and have additional training in areas pertaining to elder care.

In 2008, patients 65 years and older represented 40 percent of hospitalized adults and nearly half of all health-care dollars spent on hospitalization, but comprised less than 13 percent of the population in the United States. Individuals 85 years and older make up only 1.8 percent of the total population but account for 8 percent of every hospital discharges. Hospitalizations and health care spending for older adults are expected to rise as the population continues to age.

Just as children are not simply tiny adults, the elderly are not simply older versions of young adults. Like children, the elderly require special approaches and an understanding of the physiologic, psychosocial, and physiologic impact of aging. Evaluation of the elderly patient must focus on (1) what the patient can do, relative to what the patient should be able or wishes to do; and (2) identification of recent functional deficits that may be reversible.

Evaluation of the elderly usually differs from a standard medical evaluation. For elderly patients, especially those who are very old or frail, history-taking and physical examination may have to be done at different times, and physical examination may require two sessions because patients become fatigued. The elderly also have different, often more complicated health care problems, such as multiple disorders, which may require the use of many drugs. The emphasis in providing health care to the elderly should be on maintaining functional capabilities. Most older citizens live in the community and are intellectually intact and fully independent in their daily activities.

The population of older Americans is exploding, but there's a shortage of the very doctors trained specifically to treat them, according to the American Geriatrics Society. Geriatricians are board-certified physicians (usually family doctors or internists) with special training and certification in the health needs of older people.

"Not every older adult needs a geriatrician or will be able to find one," says Annette Medina-Walpole, M.D., chief of the division of geriatrics and aging and professor of medicine at the University of Rochester Medical Center. However, the specialists can be critical, she notes, for "people whose health conditions are causing impairment or frailty and whose family and friends feel stressed out or overwhelmed by complicated treatment plans or the need to consult multiple doctors for numerous health conditions. There are currently 7,293 certified geriatricians in the U.S. To adequately treat all the patients who would benefit most from seeing them, it would take about 20,000 of them; the American Geriatrics Society has estimated.

Yet few medical students are choosing this specialty and spots in training programs go unfilled as young doctors choose better paid fields. In 2013, just 96 residents in internal or family medicine entered a fellowship program to specialize in geriatric medicine. And it's not just doctors: Fewer than 5 percent of nurses, physician assistants, pharmacists, psychologists, and social workers have training in the unique needs of older adults. Programs across the U.S. are working to fill the gap by training more healthcare providers to treat these needs.

About 30 percent of older adults need one of these specialists, according to the American Geriatrics Society. Someone older than 75 who has several health conditions, takes a number of medications, and may also have memory loss or dementia can benefit the most from seeing a geriatrician. Geriatricians are also specially trained to look for and treat frailty: general physiological decline that often (but not always) comes with age, and can make patients more vulnerable to a litany of additional health problems.

One Dutch study found that geriatricians are more likely than general practitioners to look for early signs of frailty (such as unintentional weight loss, fatigue, and reduced strength) and more likely to address it effectively, according to another study by researchers in Spain. The specialists also routinely take a close look at the medications people take, whether they need to be adjusted, and whether age-related changes in liver and kidney function have affected how well they're working. They have particular expertise in evaluating and helping people cope with late-in-life health issues that can be overlooked or challenging to treat frailty as well as falls, incontinence, dementia, and delirium.

In a 2012 review of 50 geriatric-care studies, researchers from the Department of Veterans Affairs found that older adults who got outpatient care from a geriatrician were less likely to end up in the hospital, and their overall healthcare costs were lower.(A key focus of geriatricians is helping their patients retain autonomy. Plus those with a geriatrician as their primary-care doctor were less likely to be taking risky medications.

Investigators in New York were looking for health-care fraud hot-spots. Agents suggested Oceana, a cluster of luxury condos in Brighton Beach. The 865-unit complex had a garage full of Porsches and Aston Martins and 500 residents claiming Medicaid, which is meant for the poor, elderly and disabled. Last August six residents were charged with Medicaid fraud. Health care is a tempting target for thieves. Medicaid doles out $415 billion a year. Medicare (a federal scheme for the elderly), spends $600 billion. Total health spending in America is a massive $2.7 trillion, or 17% of GDP. No one knows for sure how much of that is embezzled.

Federal prosecutors had over 2,000 health-fraud probes open at the end of 2013. A Medicare "strike force," which was formed in 2007, boasts of seven nationwide "takedowns." In the latest, on May 13th, 90 people, including 16 doctors, were rounded up in six cities more than half of them in Miami, the capital city of medical fraud. One doctor is alleged to have fraudulently charged for $24m, including 1,000 power wheelchairs. Punishments have grown tougher: last year, the owner of a mental-health clinic got 30 years for false billing. Efforts to claw back stolen cash are highly cost-effective: in 2011-13 the government's main fraud-control program, run jointly by the Department of Health and Human Services (HHS) and the Department of Justice, recovered $8 for every $1 it spent.

As fraud-fighting has intensified, dodgy billing has tumbled in areas that were most prone to abuse, such as durable medical supplies and home visits. Home-health fraud such as charging for non-existent visits to give insulin injections got so bad that the CMS, which runs the programs, called a moratorium on enrolling new providers in several large cities last year. Since tighter screening was introduced under Obamacare, the CMS has stripped 17,000 providers of their license to bill Medicare. Thousands of suppliers also quit after being required to seek accreditation and to post surety bonds of $50,000. However, the sheer volume of transactions makes it easier for miscreants to hide: every day, for instance, Medicare's contractors process 4.5m claims. In this context the $4.3 billion recovered by fraud-busters in 2013, though a record, looks paltry.

One older popular scam: was over billing for HIV infusion, an outdated therapy that Medicare still covers despite the existence of cheaper, better alternatives. This scam waned in Florida after a crackdown, only to pop up in Detroit, run by relatives of the original perpetrators. Fraud mutates, too. As old hustles are rumbled, fraudsters invent new ones. Thousands of bogus equipment suppliers registered to empty shopfronts are decreasing. Scams now need to be more sophisticated to succeed. Doctors, pharmacies, and patients act in league. Scammers over-bill for real services rather than charging for non-existent ones. That makes them harder to spot.

Some criminals are switching from cocaine trafficking to prescription-drug fraud because the risk-adjusted rewards are higher: the money is still good, the work safer and the penalties lighter. Medicare gumshoes in Florida regularly find stockpiles of weapons when making arrests.

Stealing patients' identities is profitable as well. Medical records are worth more to criminals than credit-card numbers. They contain more information, and can be used to obtain prescriptions for controlled drugs. Usually, it takes victims longer to notice that their details have been pinched. The Government Accountability Office has recommended that the CMS remove Social Security numbers from Medicare cards to prevent fraud. It has yet to do so. In one fast-growing area of fraud, involving pharmacies and prescription drugs, federal investigators have seen caseloads quadruple over the past five years. Elderly patients may receive kickbacks to sell their details to a pharmacist. He will then provide them with drugs they need while billing Medicare for costlier ones.

Paid recruiters scour nursing homes for accomplices. Some pharmacies also pay wholesalers to produce phony invoices. Others bribe medical workers for leftover pills: in April, a pharmacy-owner in Louisiana admitted to paying nursing-home staff a few hundred dollars a time to bring her unused drugs, which she repackaged and sold as new, billing Medicare $2.2m for the recycled medications between 2008 and 2013.

Another scam is to turn a doctor's clinic into a prescription-writing factory for painkillers and resell them on the street. A clinic in New York was recently charged with fraudulently producing prescriptions for more than 5m oxycodone tablets, which were sold locally for $30-$90 each. The alleged conspirators included doctors and traffickers who ran crews of "patients" so large that long lines sometimes formed outside the clinic. The doctors charged $300 per large prescription. The fake patients typically obtained these from the traffickers at the clinic door.

Dozens of operators of ambulances and ambulettes (vans designed to take wheelchairs) have been caught offering kickbacks to patients to pretend they can't walk. This lets them qualify for "emergency" pick-ups, for which the company can charge $400 per patient.

Florida's Agency for Health Care Administration (AHCA) has recovered up to $50m a year solely from hospitals billing for treatment of illegal aliens that is wrongly coded as "emergency care." However, the work is labor-intensive. A bigger worry is that, as ever more Medicare and Medicaid beneficiaries move to "managed care" (privately administered) plans, government sleuths will have access to less data. This could lead to lower fraud-related recoveries. Efforts have been made to improve information-sharing between government and private insurers, including the creation of a public-private forum, the National Health Care Anti-Fraud Association (NHCAA).

The NCHAA is pushing for federal immunity guarantees for insurers that share fraud-related information. On May 20th, a bipartisan group of senators introduced a bill to make it easier for insurers to share data with Medicare. It would also require Medicare to check new providers for links to firms that have previously swindled the taxpayer (which you might have thought it was already doing). Obamacare has had a big impact, says Shantanu Agrawal of the CMS. One thing it requires is that when a state kicks out a dodgy Medicaid provider, it shares that information with Medicare, and vice versa. Previously, there were legal impediments to doing this, for some reason.

Elderly abuse by medical professionals can easily take place in pharmacies. Medicare fraud occurs if a pharmacy provides a generic medicine but bills for a name brand one. Fraudulent medical billing also happens when pharmacists substitute more expensive capsules in place of prescribed tablets to increase Medicare or Medicaid reimbursement. (Chicago Tribune) In another type of elder medical fraud, pharmacists charge for a certain amount of pills but dispense a lesser amount.

Elderly abuse by medical professionals furthermore, takes place in medical supply companies as well. Medicare fraud might involve illegal billing practices such as charging for a motorized wheelchair but actually providing a cheaper model. Another form of fraudulent medical billing occurs when companies fail to pick up equipment on time and continue to charge Medicare. Elder medical fraud by supply companies, like all medical fraud, can easily hurt seniors for instance, if a used or unsafe scooter is substituted for a new, high quality one.

Elderly abuse by medical professionals doesn't stop with elder abuse by doctors, pharmacists and equipment suppliers. Medicare fraud can also involve professional elder caregivers. Home health workers commit fraudulent medical billing by claiming to provide more care hours than they actually do. You can also find elder medical fraud and elderly abuse by hospital medical staff, for instance, when lab workers bill for phantom x-rays.

To cut down on elderly abuse by medical professionals, the government employs a Health Care Fraud Prevention and Enforcement Action Team, according to the U.S. Department of Health and Human Services. The team includes a Medicare Fraud Strike Force, which investigates this type of elderly abuse by healthcare professionals. Team members uncover fraudulent medical billing and report Medicare fraud. Elder medical fraud perpetrators can be arrested and, if found guilty, go to prison and/or pay heavy fines.

The 2010 report contains citations of dozens of violations committed by dozens of various health care facilities for mentally and developmentally disabled persons, as well as senior citizens. Health care fraud is not a victimless crime. Whether it's a pharmaceutical company caught over-charging Medicare for a drug, or a private physician lining his books with patient services he couldn't possibly have had time or resources to perform, we all pay in the end because anyone whoever's worked a day has paid into Social Security, and therefore, into Medicare.

The wheelchair scam was designed to exploit blind spots in Medicare, which often pays insurance claims without checking them first. Criminals disguised themselves as medical-supply companies. They made up bogus bills, saying they'd provided expensive wheelchairs to Medicare patients who, in reality, didn't need wheelchairs. They asked Medicare to pay them back, so they could pocket the huge markup that the government paid on each chair. Since 1999, Medicare has spent $8.2 billion to procure power wheelchairs and "scooters" for 2.7 million people. Today, the government cannot even guess at how much of that money was paid out to scammers.

Health care giant Johnson & Johnson and its subsidiaries have agreed to pay over $2.2 billion to resolve criminal and civil allegations of promoting three prescription drugs for off-label uses not approved by the Food and Drug Administration, the Department of Justice announced. The allegations include paying kickbacks to physicians and pharmacies to recommend and prescribe Risperdal and Invega, both antipsychotic drugs, and Natrecor, which is used to treat heart failure. "J&J's promotion of Risperdal for unapproved uses threatened the most vulnerable populations of our society - children, the elderly and those with developmental disabilities.

This action is the latest example of regulators cracking down on aggressive pharmaceutical marketing tactics, namely trying to increase sales by pushing medicines for unapproved, or "off-label," uses. While doctors are allowed to prescribe medicines for any use, drug makers cannot promote them in any way that is not approved by FDA.

The government's criminal complaint over Risperdal charged that from 2002 to 2003, sales representatives of J&J subsidiary Janssen Pharmaceuticals promoted the antipsychotic to physicians and other prescribers who treated elderly dementia patients by urging them to use the drug to treat symptoms such as anxiety, agitation, depression, hostility and confusion despite the drug only being approved to treat schizophrenia at that time. Sales reps were allegedly offered incentives for off-label promotion of the drug.

Health care consumers need to identify these health care fraudsters and report them to attempt to salvage the health care system. People need to remember that he/she could receive a monetary reward for being a whistle blower.

Whistle blowers are people who expose unethical or illegal wrongdoing within companies by reporting it internally to superiors or externally to the media, government authorities, or specialized attorneys. They can be either current or past employees (insiders), or outside individuals who are familiar with the unlawful conduct, and are

not required to be U.S. citizens. If you properly report Medicare fraud, you may be entitled to a significant whistleblower reward.

35. Infectious Disease Fraud

Many common infections can be treated by your personal physician. Infectious disease specialists diagnose and treat conditions resulting from all types of infections. These can include infections caused by bacteria, viruses, fungi and parasites. Your doctor may refer you to an infectious disease specialist if the infection is difficult to diagnose, accompanied by a high fever or does not respond to treatment.

Infectious disease (ID) specialists see patients suffering from but not limited to: Blastomycosis, Bone and joint infections, Complicated urinary tract infections, Heart valve infections, HIV/AIDS, Lyme disease, Malaria and other tropical diseases, Measles, Mumps and Rubella,, Meningitis, Methicillin-resistant Staphylococcus aureus (MRSA), Pneumonia, Post-operative infections, Rheumatic fever, Tick-borne infections, Travel Medicine and Tuberculosis. An ID specialist has 4 years of medical school, 3 years training as a doctor of internal medicine and 2-3 years specialized training in infectious diseases.

Your doctor might refer you to an ID specialist when an infection is difficult to diagnose, or an infection is accompanied by a high fever, or a patient does not respond to treatment, or a healthy person plans to travel to a foreign country or a location where infection risk is higher, or when treating illnesses becomes a part of a patient's overall care, for example, a patient with HIV/AIDS. In all of these cases, the specialized training and diagnostic tools of the ID specialist can help determine the cause of an infection and the best approach to treatment. ID specialists review the medical data, including X-rays and laboratory reports such as blood work and culture data. They also may perform a physical exam to help determine the cause of the problem.

ID specialists often order laboratory tests to examine samples of blood or other body fluids or cultures from wounds. A blood serum analysis can help the ID specialist detect antibodies that indicate what type of infection you have. These advanced tests can further explain the results of earlier tests, helping to pinpoint the problem.

Treatments consist of medicines usually antibiotics to treat the infection and prevent it from returning. These medicines may be given orally (in the form of pills or liquids) or administered directly into veins, via an IV tube. Many ID specialists have IV antibiotic therapy available in their offices, which decreases the likelihood that a patient will need to be hospitalized.

Infections are caused by infectious agents, including viruses, viroids, prions, bacteria, nematodes such as parasitic roundworms and pinworms, arthropods such as ticks, mites, fleas, and lice, fungi such as ringworm, and other macro parasites such as tapeworms and other helminths. Most infectious disease doctors acknowledge that Borrelia burgdorferi, the bacterium that causes Lyme disease, can stay in the body for years, most believe that a short course of antibiotics is enough to wipe out the infection. However, an increasingly vocal group of patients, advocates, and doctors believes the bacteria can remain within the body and persist even after treatment, causing vague symptoms. They argue that a cure requires not weeks but months or years of strong antibiotics, and that relapses are common.

A study found that people who have been treated for Lyme disease and then later appear to relapse are typically suffering from a new infection. That's not to say that everyone who claims to have chronic Lyme has had multiple infections. In a review article published by Paul Lantos, he identified seven studies conducted in endemic areas that included nearly 2,000 patients with suspected Lyme disease. Most of these patients had either an alternative medical diagnosis or a functional somatic syndrome such as chronic fatigue syndrome or fibromyalgia.

Examples of fraud and abuse include in infectious disease included: A provider discontinues privately purchasing vaccine for patients whose insurance covers immunizations and gives every patient in the practice state supplied vaccine, whether they are eligible or not. A provider bills Medicaid for administration reimbursement when no vaccines were given, A provider administers state supplied vaccine to a child, then bills the child's insurance company for the cost of the vaccine or A provider charges the patient for state supplied vaccine.

The New York State Department of Health has opened an investigation of the California laboratory, GeneX Inc. after receiving eight complaints from doctors and patients who said its Lyme tests also gave them positive results not confirmed by other labs' results. The concern about Lyme testing goes beyond New York State. This year the Food and Drug Administration and the Centers for Disease Control and Prevention released a warning about Lyme tests "whose accuracy and clinical usefulness have not been adequately established."

Guidelines from the disease control agency recommend Lyme testing only when patients have symptoms and live within an area of the United States where ticks are known to be infected with Borrelia burgdorferi, the organism that causes the disease. Under the guidelines, laboratories should first conduct a test called Elisa. But the Elisa test often gives a false-positive result, so the agency also calls for a second, more sensitive test, the Western blot.

Nationally, reported cases of Lyme disease have more than doubled in a decade, to at least 23,963 in 2003 (the most-recent year for which statistics are available) from fewer than 9,000 in 1993. Infectious disease experts agree that infections have been on the rise, but they worry that part the increase may be due to over diagnosis. A Topeka physician who lost his license, and two California residents are charged with creating a fraudulent marketing scheme to sell medical equipment and drug treatments for a nonexistent epidemic of Lyme disease.

An individual was arrested for alleged workers' compensation fraud. She worked for the Los Angeles County Department of Parks and Recreation for over 10 years at the Placerita Canyon Nature Center in Newhall handling variety of animals, including owls, skunks, reptiles and opossums. She reported that she had been bitten by a tick, contracted Lyme disease and as a result filed a workers' compensation claim with a date of injury of April 19, 2007.

A 25-count federal indictment charges the conspirators with violating the federal Food, Drug and Cosmetic Act by conspiring to sell a microscope that supposedly would diagnose Lyme disease and drugs that supposedly would cure the disease. Marketing materials claimed that Lyme disease was "the plague of the 21st century" and was a contributing factor in 50 percent of all chronic illnesses, including Chronic Fatigue Syndrome.

A California man recently pleaded guilty in Kansas City to conspiracy to commit mail fraud and to introduce "misbranded" drugs into interstate commerce. This individual, along with three co-conspirators, apparently made more than $400,000 selling a microscope via mail order that they claimed could diagnose Lyme disease, a bacterial illness contracted from tick bites. They even reportedly claimed to have a treatment plan to cure the disease, which can cause flu-like symptoms and could develop into abnormalities in the joints, heart and nervous system.

Hard enough as it is to believe, the 79-year-old defendant and his cohorts thought they could get away with the scam, which is until their product caused one person to go into a coma and die and caused a renal failure in another. After the tragedies came to light, authorities discovered that this company, American Biologics, was not registered with the FDA to produce drugs or medical devices.

Some self-anointed LLMD's (Lyme-Literate Medical Doctors) have jumped on the bandwagon of "chronic Borrelia neurotoxins" and are insisting upon the need to "detoxify" them. Since there exists no solid evidence for the existence of such toxins, their treatment guidelines are bogus. The myth started with patent application, and they claim ownership to any diagnostic/treatment process based on their discovery of a coding sequence in the Bb genome for a toxin they say is similar to Botulin C2 toxin, calling it BbTox1. The presence of genes is no guarantee for the actual expression of those genes.

Until the existence of Lyme neurotoxins is proven the "detoxifiers" and "toxin binders" such as Cholestyramine (Questran) have never proven their value in any randomized, double-blind, placebo-controlled, peer-reviewed, reproducible trial, but they do have very serious potential side effects, including cancer.

The big issues impeding a speedy resolution of symptoms under treatment are antibiotic resistance, bacterial persistence and excessive immune reactions to relatively low bacterial loads. Neuro-Lyme patients need open-ended antibiotic treatment with high doses of appropriate antibiotic combinations.

Several doctors who market themselves as "Lyme specialists" have been disciplined by state medical boards for unprofessional conduct. The activist network is seeking laws to block further board action against such doctors. In line with this, the Romney flier advocates providing "local physicians with protection from lawsuits to ensure they can treat the disease with the aggressive antibiotics that are required."

In 2009, a practitioner in New Mexico, was charged with fraud in connection with diagnosing and treating people for Lyme disease. The criminal complaint stated: This individual represented to patients whom he has cured 100% of the 3,000 people he claims to have treated for Lyme disease. He makes his diagnoses after examining a blood specimen with a Bradford Variable Projection High Resolution Microscope, a device not approved by the FDA for diagnosing any medical condition.

The purported treatment is an intravenous cocktail that contains dioxychlor and sulfoxine substances that lack FDA approval for any purpose. Patients typically pay about $5,000 for these services. Dioxychlor, sulfoxine, and the microscope system were marketed by American Biologics, a company that had sold questionable products for more than 30 years.

The company claimed that Dioxychlor was "a natural antibiotic that kills bacteria by supplying generous amounts of oxygen to organisms that do not require oxygen for growth and may even die in its presence." In 2006, Health Canada advised against the use of these products and the Bradford microscope.

Health care consumers need to identify these health care fraudsters and report them to attempt to salvage the health care system. People need to remember that he/she could receive a monetary reward for being a whistle blower.

Whistle blowers are people who expose unethical or illegal wrongdoing within companies by reporting it internally to superiors or externally to the media, government authorities, or specialized attorneys. They can be either current or past employees (insiders), or outside individuals who are familiar with the unlawful conduct, and are not required to be U.S. citizens. If you properly report Medicare fraud, you may be entitled.

36. Internal Medicine Fraud

Internal medicine or general medicine as defined by Wikipedia is the medical specialty dealing with the prevention, diagnosis, and treatment of adult diseases. Physicians specializing in internal medicine are called internists or physicians in Commonwealth nations. Internists are skilled in the management of patients who have undifferentiated or multi-system disease processes. Internists care for hospitalized and ambulatory patients and may play a major role in teaching and research.

Peninsula Internal Medicine, was closed Wednesday while federal agents seized medical records as part of their investigation into whether or not the practice had fraudulently billed Medicare and Medicaid for almost $1 million over an eight-year period. The investigators were assigned with the U.S. Department of Health and Human Services, Office of Inspector General, a law enforcement agency tasked with investigating fraud and abuse of the two programs, along with 100 others provided by the department.

What passersby and turned away patients didn't know on June 29 is that federal investigators were jamming a box truck full of patient records, invoices, bills, audits and computers in an effort to find evidence supporting the fraud allegations. Peninsula Internal, according to the affidavit, had billed the practice for bloodwork it didn't perform; smoking cessation counseling for nonsmokers and for services rendered on Fridays by the doctor on a day he did not work, according to documents from the U.S. Attorney's Office made available to The Daily Times on Thursday.

Four people are charged for mass-marketing a talking glucose monitor and sending the devices to Medicare patients across the country who didn't need or request them. They billed Medicare for the devices and received more than $22 million. In some cases health care providers paid kickbacks to fraudsters who could get their hands on Medicare patients' personal information. They would then use that info to bill Medicare for bogus care.

Sometimes fraudsters, known to the Feds as "patient recruiters," will go to places like homeless shelters and soup kitchens and offer money to those who would share their Medicare patient numbers, a Department of Justice spokesman said.

A Los Angeles doctor is charged for allegedly billing $23 million for 1,000 power wheelchairs and home health services that were not medically necessary and often not provided. And in a Florida case, a health care provider received $1.6 million from Medicare for prescription drugs that were never purchased and never dispensed, said Lynch. A Las Vegas-based internal medicine group has agreed to pay $300,000 to resolve civil allegations of healthcare fraud, according to a Las Vegas Review Journal report. The physician group allegedly billed Medicare and the Federal Employee Health Benefits Program for cholesterol tests that were medically unnecessary between Jan. 2003 and Dec. 2006, according to the report.

In order to get paid, doctors have to label everything they do for a patient with a billing code. Routine visits for established patients are billed on a scale of 1 to 5. A level 1 code is for a short, easy office visit; level 5 is meant for the longest, most complicated office visits, which are also paid at a higher rate. Office visits account for about $12 billion in Medicare spending every year.

Three California physicians are among the top five nationally in billing for the highest number of complex, "level 5" office visits. Nationwide, some 1,800 doctors always billed at the highest level possible for routine office visits. In Colorado, 71 doctors billed at the highest possible level for every one of their Medicare office visits.

An internist, had nothing to say as he stood before a County Circuit Court Judge for sentencing. The judge suspended the 30 days in jail called for in the Michigan Sentencing Guidelines but imposed 250 hours of community service. He must pay restitution to Blue Cross of $694. Branch County Assistant Prosecuting Attorney Chris Anderson suggested the doctor might see people who are abusing the type of drug he prescribed. The doctor's trouble began when he wrote a prescription for 180 OxyContin to his office manager, which was billed to the office managers Blue Cross health insurance. The prescription was for a patientwho did not have insurance.

Anderson said the circumstances "might almost seem noble but we are dealing with a controlled substance that is highly abused in this community." The prosecutor noted there are people who obtain pain medication prescriptions to sell on the streets.

Health care consumers need to identify these health care fraudsters and report them to attempt to salvage the health care system. People need to remember that he/she could receive a monetary reward for being a whistle blower.

Whistle blowers are people who expose unethical or illegal wrongdoing within companies by reporting it internally to superiors or externally to the media, government authorities, or specialized attorneys. They can be either current or past employees (insiders), or outside individuals who are familiar with the unlawful conduct, and are not required to be U.S. citizens. If you properly report Medicare fraud, you may be entitled.

37. Kidney Disease Fraud

Nephrology is a specialty of medicine and pediatrics that concerns itself with the study of normal kidney function, kidney problems, the treatment of kidney problems and renal replacement therapy (dialysis and kidney transplantation). Nephrologists are medical doctors who specialize in the diagnosis and treatment of diseases of the kidney and urinary system, such as inflammation of the kidneys, chronic kidney disease, or cancer.

Nephrologists may further specialize in treating certain age groups, such as pediatric nephrologists, who only treat children. Nephrologists may consult with people for short-term illnesses or procedures, such as for a kidney biopsy, or they may serve as a primary doctor for people who have long-term (chronic) kidney problems or who are on dialysis. Nephrologists can be board-certified in nephrology through the Board of Internal Medicine, which is recognized by the American Board of Medical Specialties Urologists are medical doctors who specialize in the diagnosis and treatment of diseases of the urinary system in men and women and disorders of the male reproductive system.

Like some other physicians, nephrologists occasionally commit medical fraud. A former Washington state kidney doctor could face prison time and millions of dollars in fines if convicted of overbilling the federal government and private insurance companies. After hearing secret testimony, a federal grand jury returned a 14-count indictment against a nephrologist and his corporation.

He is accused of masterminding a scheme to defraud Medicare, Medicaid and private insurance companies of at least $1.5 million over five years. This doctor would have to repay the money he's accused of bilking from insurers. He also faces up to $3.5 million in fines and 70 years in prison, although that length of sentence is unlikely. The indictment caps a fraud investigation that lasted more than 2 years. The doctor is accused of asking other doctors in the group to bill insurers for a higher level of inpatient care than patients needed for two major types of dialysis. This type of fraud is called "up coding.""

The doctor in question is accused of systematically filing false insurance claims for services not necessary or not documented. He allegedly asked other doctors in the group to make two progress notes on the records of hospitalized patients receiving two types of kidney dialysis- hemodialysis and peritoneal dialysis because an inpatient visit billed with two notes pays a doctor significantly more than an inpatient visit billed with one note.

A medical director at dialysis clinics in Georgia was discussing clinic procedures with one of the nurses. The two men say they saw something they believed was very wrong: expensive medicine, and lots of it, was being tossed in the trash. And the clinic workers were being told to do it, the two men say. The alleged waste was being carried out on a massive scale and the nurse and the doctor said, they knew why almost immediately. They claim it was a way for their company, DaVita Inc., to defraud the government, over bill Medicare and Medicaid and make a fortune. The profit this company raked from those two schemes, only from those two drugs, was hundreds of millions of dollars."

The two individuals said the alleged fraud schemes they discovered were going on at the company's clinics all across the country with tens of thousands of patients. It was a deliberate strategy coordinated by the company. It was just a scheme in order to fraudulently increase and maximize and boost the Medicare revenue, Medicare payment, so therefore fraudulently increase their revenue. DaVita Inc., based in downtown Denver, is one of the nation's largest dialysis companies. DaVita has grown in the past couple of years and now runs roughly 2,000 dialysis clinics across the country, which has added up to a $7 billion business. The head of the company is reportedly paid an estimated $15 million a year, according to the Wall Street Journal, which has called him the best compensated CEO in Colorado. Most of DaVita's revenue came from Medicare and Medicaid payments.

If the allegations are true, the company threw away hundreds of millions of dollars of medicine, and taxpayers paid for it. And, if true, the alleged fraud schemes could represent one of the largest Medicare frauds in U.S. history. DaVita instructed its nurses to administer a 100-milligram dose of the iron drug Venofor. For example, if a patient requires this dose once per week, you'd administer 100 milligrams, waste nothing and charge Medicare for 100 milligrams.

DaVita , instead of a chargpng for one vial, they give 50 milligrams of this vial and)put the residual into the trash. With another vial, the company would give 25 milligrams to a patient and put the rest in the trash, then repeat it with yet another vial, when one vial could have been given without waste. The more vials DaVita used, the more the company was able to bill the government, the men say. Two individuals claim they tried to call attention to the massive waste and tried to get it stopped. But instead, they say, they were basically told to stop causing trouble and to continue following the companies protocols.

One of the physician employees quit his job and left the clinic rather than continue where fraud was going on. The other employee claimed the company punished him for speaking up. Of course, once they found out, they did not renew my medical directorship or my practice the doctor employee claimed. "We are a three-physician practice, and it was a significant loss of revenue.

Today, both men have filed a whistle blower lawsuit under the U.S. False Claims Act on behalf of the U.S. government, charging DaVita with massive Medicare fraud. They stand to make millions if DaVita is found guilty. But other companies, including DaVita's main competitor, used smaller vials and smaller combinations at times, limiting what was thrown away.

A settlement was finalized recently by a local nephrology physician practice group, and certain affiliated dialysis centers in Tennessee. A medical group agreed to pay $4.36 million to settle alleged violations of the Federal False Claims Act, the Tennessee Medicaid False Claims Act, and other federal and state laws and regulations.

A government investigation revealed that from at least 2001 through 2006, the medical group submitted numerous false and fraudulent claims to government health programs, including Medicare and TennCare, for payment through a pattern of up coding for various physician services.

Most kidney dialysis patients are anemic. Epogen, made by Amgen, is commonly used in dialysis clinics to boost patients' red blood cell counts back to healthy levels. Medicare pays the bills of long-term dialysis patients. A Texas whistle blower lawsuit accused DaVita of using more Epogen than was medically necessary, and for double-billing the government for Epogen left over in vials and reused. For the period covered by the lawsuit, the payment system rewarded dialysis companies by reimbursing for the amount of drugs used, critics have said.

Medicare payments for dialysis cost the US government $5 billion a year. The global market for chronic dialysis services is worth approximately $43 billion, and the US market is the largest in the world in terms of value. Worldwide, by the end of 2005, the number of dialysis patients reached 1.5 million. Of that number, approximately 23% patients were treated in the US, 20 percent in Europe, 17% in Japan, and 40% in the rest of the world.

The 6th largest medical fraud case in US history was settled in December 2004 against Gambro Healthcare for $325 million. At the time, Gambro was the third largest operator of renal-dialysis clinics in the US. The settlement period covered fraud that occurred from January 1, 1991 through September 30, 2004. Gambro Healthcare is owned by a holding company, Gambro Inc., a subsidiary of Gambro AB, headquartered in Stockholm, Sweden, which produces dialysis products, operates dialysis clinics and markets blood bank technology products. In fiscal 2004, the company had revenue of $3.6 billion. Gambro had revenue of $1.4 billion in the first nine months of 2005, with the latter significantly lower than 2004 due to the company selling off its US operations to DaVita in October 2005.

The federal fraud investigation began in 2001, after a nephrologist filed a federal whistle blower lawsuit against the company in St. Louis, alleging fraudulent billing practices. The nephrologist served as Gambro's chief medical officer from 1995 to 2000, according to the lawsuit complaint.On December 2, 2004, the Department of Justice announced that Gambro would pay a significant fine. At least four separate class-action lawsuits have been filed against DaVita Healthcare over the use of Granuflo and Naturalyte at the company's dialysis centers, which have been linked to an increased risk of cardiac arrest and sudden death during hemodialysis treatment.

The two dialysis products were manufactured and sold by Fresenius Medical Care, and they were widely used at DaVita dialysis clinics throughout the United States before being recalled, according to the lawsuits.

NaturaLyte is a liquid acid concentrate, and GranuFlo is a dry acid concentrate. Both products contain sodium acetate that allegedly converts to bicarbonate at higher-than-expected levels for most doctors. A recall for Granuflo and NaturaLyte was issued by Fresenius Medical

Care in early 2012, after a warning was issued about the risks associated with the products and the importance of doctors monitoring bicarbonate levels during treatment.

Fresenius Medical Care not only manufactures and sells the dialysis products, but also owns and operates thousands of dialysis clinics throughout the United States that directly compete with DaVita clinics. In late 2011, an internal review of patients treated at 667 Fresenius clinics found at least 941 instances where patients suffered a cardiac arrest during dialysis treatment. To furthermore, demonstrate greed in the medical profession a surgeon with close ties to the Bay Area was charged with prescribing excessive drugs to a comatose, disabled patient to hasten his death and harvest his organs for transplantation for patients with severe kidney disease.

Health care consumers need to identify these health care fraudsters and report them to attempt to salvage the health care system. People need to remember that he/she could receive a monetary reward for being a whistle blower.

Whistle blowers are people who expose unethical or illegal wrongdoing within companies by reporting it internally to superiors or externally to the media, government authorities, or specialized attorneys. They can be either current or past employees (insiders), or outside individuals who are familiar with the unlawful conduct, and are not required to be U.S. citizens. If you properly report Medicare fraud, you may be entitled.

38. Neurology Fraud

Neurology as defined by Wikipedia is a branch of medicine dealing with disorders of the nervous system. Neurology deals with the diagnosis and treatment of all categories of conditions and disease involving the central and peripheral nervous system (and its subdivisions, the autonomic nervous system and the somatic nervous system); including their coverings, blood vessels, and all effector tissue, such as muscle.

A Tennessee neurologist was arraigned in federal court in Detroit on Tuesday, May 6, on charges of health care fraud and distribution of controlled substances. The FBI, Drug Enforcement Administration and Internal Revenue Service are investigating this neurologist saying he prescribed unneeded medication to patients and billed Medicare and private insurers for tests he didn't conduct. In a five-year period, he collected six times as much money from Medicare than the nearest U.S. prescriber of a controlled drug to treat cancer pain, according to a May 2 affidavit from a federal investigator. The conditions of his bond state he cannot prescribe controlled substances, bill Medicare or other federal health care programs and must surrender his concealed pistol license and passport.

Medicare paid a neurologist $6.9 million from Jan. 1, 2009, through Feb. 6, 2014, for Subsys he prescribed. The next highest amount a U.S. prescriber received was $1.6 million. He is responsible for approximately 20.3 percent of the Subsys prescribed to Medicare beneficiaries nationwide during this time," the affidavit stated. He wrote 1,283 prescriptions for the drug in five years, while the next closest prescriber wrote 203 prescriptions, the complaint stated. Subsys is an opioid used to relieve chemotherapy-induced nausea and pain. The Food and Drug Administration requires the drug be prescribed through a management program because of the risk for addiction, abuse and overdose, the affidavit stated. This neurologist also collected more than $5 million in the past five years by billing insurers for procedures he did not conduct, such as nerve conduction studies and needle electromyographies, the affidavit states.

Undercover police officers visited him seven times from April 2011 to May 2013. For those visits, Awerbuch collected $4,973.08

from Blue Cross, Blue Shield of Michigan for the procedures and treatments, according to the affidavit. Officers, who visually recorded treatments, reported the neurologist did not sterilize the needle for the needle electromyography treatment or wipe down the patient's leg or foot prior to treatment, nor did the officers receiving treatment report feeling electric shock during the two- to three-minute treatments. According to the affidavit, a neurologist who specializes in such treatments said the neurologist in question could not have conducted the exams because they generally take 20 to 90 minutes.

On one visit, an undercover officer asked for a Vicodin prescription and attempted to bribe the neurologist for the drug with $1,000. The officer told the neurologist, he would sell the drug to coworkers. The neurologist refused the bribe and asked the officer not to sell Vidodin again. He also asked if the officer was a Drug Enforcement Administration for FBI agent. The officer said he was not, and the neurologist him the Vicodin prescription. During a later visit, the neurologist prescribed Subsys to the officer even though the officer had not been diagnosed with cancer.

A Yonkers neurologist is among six people accused of running a $57 million health care scam, officials said. Another neurologist is facing federal criminal charges for his role in submitting false insurance claims, the U.S. Attorney's Office announced on Wednesday. He is also facing a civil lawsuit that was filed by a whistle blower in 2015 and was unsealed on Wednesday, officials said. Officials said between 2003 and November 2015 the operation centered on City Medical Associates, a cardiology and neurology clinic in the Queens. Employees at CMA allegedly submitted phony claims to insurance providers, including providers paid through Medicaid and Medicare, by lying that medical tests had been ordered or performed by doctors who did not work at CMA.

The neurologist allegedly participated in the fraud by allowing CMA to submit false claims to insurance providers under his name. Bogus claims were also submitted under the names of two other doctors who did not know that their identities were being used for the scam, officials said. The doctor worked part-time for CMA between 2002 and 2004, and from 2008 until 2015, he helped the crew fraudulently bill insurance providers for about $57 million, according to the federal indictment. The phony claims referenced medical tests that were never ordered or performed, according to the indictment.

From at least 2012 until November 2015, the neurologist allegedly allowed CMA to use his name for the scheme in exchange for CMA providing him with health insurance coverage at no cost, even though he was not a CMA employee at that time. On June 28, 2016, the doctor lied to an FBI special agent when he said he had not dealt with CMA since his employment there ended in 2004, according to the indictment. Many of the patients seen by the accused CMA employees were referred there by doctors who received kickbacks from those CMA employees, according to the indictment. The doctor faces charges of conspiracy to commit health care fraud and wire fraud, health care fraud, wire fraud, making false statements relating to health care matters, conspiracy to commit fraud in connection with identification information, and making false statements to a federal agent.

A Charlotte neurologist has agreed to pay $2 million-plus interest to the United States to settle civil fraud allegations. is the owner of and principal neurologist at The Neurological Institute in Charlotte, formerly known as Neurological Consultants of the Carolinas. The settlement was reached following a multi-year investigation by HHS-OIG into the neurologist's practices associated with the administration of intravenous immunoglobulin (IVIG) therapy.

Government investigators found that from October 13, 2003 to May 26, 2006, the doctor failed to meet the Medicare supervision regulations associated with IVIG therapy. IVIG is the delivery of healthy immunoglobulins directly into the bloodstream of patients suffering from immunodeficiency and autoimmune disorders. IVIG therapy involves the injection of a thick, viscous fluid into the veins of patients throughout a period of several hours. The Medicare program requires that the patient's physician directly supervise the administration of this treatment in order to ensure the safety of the patient. Investigators found that the doctor sought and obtained reimbursement for his IVIG therapy services from Medicare even though he was not present in the building with his patients when they were receiving IVIG treatment, as required by Medicare.

The Settlement Agreement also requires that the neurologist in question pay an additional $500,000 to Medicare upon the sale of his real estate holdings. Furthermore, this neurologist entered into a five-year Integrity Agreement with HHS-OIG to promote compliance with the statutes, regulations, program requirements, and written directives of Medicare, Medicaid, and all other federal health care programs.

"This doctor allowed his staff to practice a potentially hazardous procedure on Medicare patients, without his supervision, then blatantly charge taxpayers," said Derrick Jackson of the HHS-OIG region, including North Carolina. "Citizens of this State can continue to look toward U.S. Attorney Tompkins to vigorously pursue providers who shortcut Medicare regulations in exchange for profit."

The investigation and charges are the work of the Western District's joint Health Care Fraud Task Force. The Task Force is a multi-agency team of experienced federal and state investigators, working in conjunction with criminal and civil Assistant United States Attorneys, dedicated to identifying and prosecuting those who defraud the health care system, and reducing the potential for health care fraud in the future. T

The Task Force focuses on the coordination of cases, information sharing, identification of trends in health care fraud throughout the region, staffing of all whistle blower complaints and the creation of investigative teams so that individual agencies may focus their unique areas of expertise on investigations. The Task Force builds upon existing partnerships between the agencies, and its work reflects a heightened effort to reduce fraud and recover taxpayer dollars.

A health system in Jacksonville, Fla., is paying $2.5 million to settle claims in a whistle-blower lawsuit that it was overpaid by Medicare because its former chief neurologist was misdiagnosing patients with multiple sclerosis and other serious diseases. The neurologist was suspended in 2013 from practicing in Florida because of allegations of sexual misconduct with a patient.

The Justice Department alleges that officials at Baptist Health, a three-hospital knew that some neurology patients had been "misdiagnosed and mistreated" from September 2009 to October 2011, and the system failed to immediately tell government officials about it. Baptist Health officials said they disagree with the government's claims, including the allegation that any patient was misdiagnosed. "The claims resolved by this settlement are allegations only, and there has been no determination of liability," a statement from the system says. "Our focus remains on providing the best-quality care for our patients and their families."

Justice Department officials are attempting to decide whether to pursue allegations that the neurologist had intentionally misdiagnosed "scores" of patients with MS, brain lesions and other conditions to provide medically unnecessary services and bill for unneeded prescription drugs. Those allegations against the neurologist were included in a 2012 civil whistle-blower lawsuit. Florida's Board of Medicine suspended the doctor's medical license for one year starting in August 2013 and fined him $10,000 after he settled a complaint from the state Health Department (PDF) that he had an inappropriate sexual relationship with a female patient from August to November 2011. The neurologist had been treating the 44-year-old patient weekly for MS.

Nationally, there is a wide diversity of opinion on the diagnosis of progressive neurological conditions. Some physicians diagnose MS when early signs suggest the presence of the condition and begin treatment to slow its progression. Other physicians though choose to wait for more signs or symptoms before treating the condition, and prefer to follow criteria recommended by national MS organizations.

In January, two neurologists pleaded guilty to their roles in a scheme to pay patient recruiters illegal kickbacks for the recruitment of homeless patients. The recruited homeless patients underwent a variety of medical treatments, many of which were not medically necessary and were billed to federal healthcare programs.

A Health System in Wilmington, Del., agreed to pay $3.3 million to settle a whistle blower kickback lawsuit. In March, the health system agreed to pay $3.3 million to settle kickback allegations. According to the charges, the health system overpaid neurologists for in-hospital readings of EEGs allegedly as a "reward" for referring patients to the hospital. The court documents note the payments were part of a contract dating to 1989, prior to the enactment of the current Stark Act and Delaware Anti-kickback Statute.

The government partially joined a whistle blower (qui tam) lawsuit in Jacksonville, Florida, who alleged, among other things, that the former Chief of Neurology at a local hospital had provided unnecessary and unreasonable services to hundreds of patients, including intentionally misdiagnosing healthy patients with serious conditions such as multiple sclerosis or brain lesions, in order to bill for expensive treatment and medications. In common law, a writ of qui tam is a writ whereby a private individual who assists a prosecution can receive all or part of any penalty imposed. Many of these unnecessary services were billed to Medicare, Medicaid and other government programs and government-funded health plans, in violation of the federal False Claims Act and Florida False Claims Act.

The lawsuit was filed in January 2012 in the Middle District of Florida under the quit am, or whistleblower, provisions of the federal False Claims Act and parallel provisions of Florida's False Claims Act. These provisions permit private parties to sue on behalf of the federal and state governments and when they believe an individual or company has submitted false claims for government funds.

"We are pleased with this result as this case serves as another example of how the False Claims Act empowers Americans to help fight fraud on the government and American taxpayers, no matter how big or small the fraud may be. It demonstrates how ordinary citizens who care about following the law and doing the right thing can make a difference," said Milberg partner Kirk Chapman.

During preliminary examinations in February and April, there was testimony that Medicaid and Medicare were fraudulently billed for a procedure by another neurologist who would result in a photograph attached to the patients' charts. No such photograph was found.

The motion states that the neurologist diagnosed multiple patients with fibromyalgia and subjected them to unnecessary injections as a requirement for those patients to receive powerful narcotics. Upon investigating, a neurologist not affiliated with the case examined patients' charts and found there was no medical need for the injections. The doctor concluded the patients tolerated the injections to obtain drugs.

One of these patients said that if she objected to injections, she would not receive narcotic medications. Another patient was subject to injections 11 times between February 2011 and July 2012, according to the motion. Another patient said she was given trigger point injections in July of 2012, but a bill to Medicaid showed those injections as well as occipital nerve injections, a more expensive procedure that the patient refused. Another patient indicated that the injections caused her pain, and when she complained about them to the neurologist, she was told she would be dropped as a patient.

One patient testified that she was attending her husband's appointment when the neurologist heard she was having shoulder pain. The woman said the doctor administered occipital block injections and trigger point injections, which were billed to Medicare. She said she had not wanted the shots, and reactions to them forced her to visit the emergency room the next day.

Health care consumers need to identify these health care fraudsters and report them to attempt to salvage the health care system. People need to remember that he/she could receive a monetary reward for being a whistle blower.

Whistle blowers are people who expose unethical or illegal wrongdoing within companies by reporting it internally to superiors or externally to the media, government authorities, or specialized attorneys. They can be either current or past employees (insiders), or outside individuals who are familiar with the unlawful conduct, and are not required to be U.S. citizens. If you properly report Medicare fraud, you may be entitled to a significant whistleblower reward.

39. Neurosurgery Fraud

Neurosurgery, or neurological surgery, is the medical specialty concerned with the prevention, diagnosis, surgical treatment, and rehabilitation of disorders, which affect any portion of the nervous system, including the brain, spinal cord, peripheral nerves, and extra-cranial cerebrovascular system. In the United States, a neurosurgeon must generally complete four years of undergraduate education, four years of medical school, and seven years of residency.

Neurosurgeons like any of the other physicians mentioned throughout this book can be tempted to commit medical fraud. A neurosurgeon, for example, was accused of performing lumbar spinal fusions on numerous patients and billing insurers despite failing to install medical devices in patients whose pain continued after surgery. He is accused of using various businesses and medical practices to perpetuate the alleged fraud. The firm allegedly billed health care programs for services that were not provided or overcharged for the services, according to the criminal complaint.

In some instances, he operated on patients and dictated in his operative reports which he knew would later be used to support fraudulent insurance claims that he had performed a spinal fusion with instrumentation, when he had not. Specifically, this surgeon fraudulently billed public and private health care programs for instrumentation when, in fact, he used cortical bone dowels made of tissue. He failed to render services in relation to lumbar and thoracic fusion surgeries, including in certain instances, billing for implants that were not provided.

This surgeon admitted that, in approximately February 2010, while he was on the staff of a California hospital, he became involved with Apex Medical Technologies, which was owned by another neurosurgeon and three non-physicians. In exchange for the opportunity to invest in Apex and share in its profits, this surgeon agreed to convince his hospital to buy spinal implant devices from Apex and to use a substantial number Apex spinal implant devices in his surgical procedures. He further admitted that he, and Apex's co-owners concealed his involvement in Apex from the hospitals and surgical centers.

Another neurosurgeon in Michigan was sentenced to nearly 20 years in prison after pleading guilty to a $2.8 million health care fraud scheme in which he performed unnecessary invasive spinal surgeries. Two neurosurgeons are accused of conspiring to solicit and receive commissions from medical device manufacturers related to the purchase of spinal implants and supplies used during spinal fusion surgeries performed by these surgeons.

One neurosurgeon and his fiancée operated a business to serve as the distributors of medical devices and supplies to this neurosurgeon and his neurosurgery practice. The two are accused of demanding and getting paid exorbitant commissions by medical device manufacturers for medical devices and supplies purchased by the hospital where the surgeon performed spinal fusion surgeries. The hospital's purchases were based on the neurosurgeon's decision to use those devices and supplies during operations he performed.

According to the indictment, once the device in question was purchased by the hospital when he started operating, this surgeon generally used more spinal implants in each of his surgeries while performing more surgeries than he typically performed. In December 2008, the first full month of operation for the medical supply company, this neurosurgeon ordered about $1,330,090 worth of spinal implants for his surgeries, more than twice as much as his nearest medical peer in the local health care market. Court documents show that this neurosurgeon and his fiancée used the money they made to buy a house, a boat, an airplane, and various home improvements.

In a university hospital Medicare-fraud case a medical whistle blower alleged that clerks were ordered to forge doctor signatures and re-create old records. As in many other cases of medical fraud, pressure from authorities and fear of losing their employment, kept employees at the Medical Center's facility quiet.

Another university medical center has agreed to pay more than $2.5 million to the federal government to settle whistle blowers" claims that some of its neurosurgeons billed Medicare for participating in surgeries in which they weren't sufficiently involved, in violation of the False Claims Act. The suit in federal court alleges the neurosurgeons billed for assisting in or supervising procedures by other surgeons, residents, fellows and physician assistants that they weren't participating in to the required degree, according to the U.S.

Department of Justice. The hospital didn't admit any liability as part of the settlement.

The settlement also applies to allegations that one neurosurgeon billed Medicare for levels of spinal decompression not performed during multilevel spinal surgeries, and the university medical center has paid the federal government $840,000 to resolve allegations that it violated the False Claims Act. The medical center is alleged to have knowingly billed federal health care programs for neurosurgeries involving residents who did not receive the required level of supervision from teaching physicians.

This medical school in question employs teaching physicians who provide medical care to patients and supervise residents. The civil settlement resolves a lawsuit filed under the quit am or whistle blower provisions of the False Claims Act, which allows private citizens with knowledge of fraud to bring a civil action on behalf the United States and share in any recovery. As part of the resolution, the whistle blower will receive a share of the settlement.

The quit am complaint alleged that the university medical center submitted false claims to the Medicare and TRICARE programs for teaching physicians' services in performing neurosurgeries involving residents. If a resident helps perform a surgery, Medicare will pay for a teaching physician's service only if he/she was present in the surgery's key parts and either remained immediately available throughout the surgery or else arranged for a back-up surgeon to be available. MCW allegedly billed for teaching physicians' services even though they were responsible for multiple overlapping surgeries and did not satisfy those supervision requirements.

A Milwaukee spine surgeon has been indicted for lying to payers about minimally invasive spine procedures requiring nerve monitoring. A neurosurgeon was charged on May 16, 2013 with 13 counts of health care fraud by a federal grand jury. The neurosurgeon allegedly recruited another physician to dictate reports making it appear that the second physician had conducted interoperative nerve monitoring during surgeries performed by the neurosurgeon. According to the government, the second physician had no training or experience in, nor did he conduct intraoperative nerve monitoring during any of the surgeries.

The indictment alleges that the neurosurgeon paid the second physician $150 for each report he dictated. The neurosurgeon then used the reports prepared by the second physician to submit claims to insurance companies seeking payment for the second physician's services. According to to the indictment, the neurosurgeon submitted claims to insurance companies totaling more than $265, 000 and ultimately received approximately $82, 000. The neurosurgeon allegedly paid the second physician a total of $14, 850 for dictating the reports.

Another neurosurgeon was arrested on charges after a lengthy investigation revealed that he had taken over $50,000 in money intended for patients participating in research programs at a Spine Institute, where he was employed as a research doctor.

A Bloomfield Hills neurosurgeon allegedly defrauded the Medicare health care program for seniors of millions of dollars by performing unnecessary spinal surgeries on patients, according to a complaint unsealed Monday in federal court. This surgeon was accused of performing lumbar spinal fusions on numerous patients and billing insurers despite failing to install medical devices in patients whose pain continued after surgery.

A doctor is accusing a university hospital of retaliating against him for speaking out against what he calls dangerous medical practices, fraud and other unethical activities at the teaching hospital. In a lawsuit filed in federal court, the neurosurgeon said the hospital put profit ahead of safety by letting one doctor oversee complex spine surgery on two patients in two different operating rooms at the same time, created phony medical documents and submitted fraudulent bills to Medicare and Medicaid. The doctor, a neurosurgeon, said in the suit that when he complained about these and other issues, the hospital demoted him, cut his pay and diverted some of his cases.

A billing clerk began working as a billing specialist at a Neurosurgery office in March 2012. In 2014, the business owner, a surgeon, hired an auditor. The auditor noted resistance from the clerk, and then began reviewing books and immediately noticed red flags; clients who were not billed. After the auditor confronted this individual, she promptly resigned.

Further investigation revealed that this clerk had written herself 95 checks for more than $200,000, and used the neurosurgeon's signature stamp to endorse them. The clerk would issue checks to herself, but later change office records to show the payees as legitimate vendors of the neurosurgery clinic. In addition, this individual made

221 online purchases from company computers using the company's American Express card. The purchases were from a variety of sellers like Amazon, Macy's, Target, Lane Bryant and others, totaling more than $23,000.

A state office of professional medical conduct is probing two neurosurgeons accused of doing questionable surgery for financial gain. The doctors have been at the center of a legal and public misconduct, when a hospital suspended them for failing to show up for their patient who was anesthetized in the operating room and prepped for surgery. The hospital quietly suspended them.

A California billing company bills $38 million a year for neurosurgery services, but lawsuits charge a neurosurgeon with operating on patients unnecessarily. The chief of neurosurgery at a large center for head trauma and has been accused repeatedly of performing unnecessary surgeries, making grave errors in the operating room and lying to patients.

A specific neurosurgeon controls the most high-profile surgical service at a California medical despite 33 malpractice or wrongful-death complaints and three investigations by the Medical Board of California. This neurosurgeon moved to a medical center in 1995 after losing his teaching post at a California medical center, after receiving allegations of incompetence and poor judgment. Since then, he has been sued 10 times as often as the average neurosurgeon in his community. Five of those lawsuits say surgeries for which the surgeon billed hundreds of thousands of dollars were not medically necessary. Distressed patients and some doctors alleged that the medical center had overlooked negligent and unethical behavior by the neurosurgeon because of the revenue his department generated which as more than $38 million a year.

A former California hospital executive at the center of a $500 million kickback scheme that subjected injured workers to risky spinal surgeries is attempting to spread the blame by suing his alleged co-conspirators, according to a recent court filing. This hospital executive has identified 22 doctors, health executives, chiropractors and a lawyer, suggesting that they accepted money in exchange for running patients through his surgery suites, pharmacies and MRI machines. The lawsuit, in essence, says that if he has to pay for the alleged scam, they should, also.

Another doctor sent an injured workman's compensation patient to another neurosurgeon who said the case struck him as intriguing. He said he found it odd that both the injured worker and her surgeon were traveling 75 miles for a surgery that could have been done in a county where they both lived. He was surprised to hear that she was picked up for surgery in a white van, put up in a Long Beach-area motel and given meal vouchers. It was really unlike any surgical services I'd ever heard of before.

A Federal investigator said that while building his case, he developed a confidential tipster who told him that the hospital executive was flying the neurosurgeon in a private plane to Long Beach, California and paying him $15,000 kickbacks to do the surgeries.

The neurosurgeon in question settled his malpractice case in July 2014 for $500,000, court records show, noting that other defendants also played a role in the patient's care. The hospital executive's allegations opened a new chapter in a case of corruption that reached to the highest levels of California state government, even as it pulled poor Latino workers out of the Central Valley to stud their spines with overpriced surgical hardware. The hospital executive pleaded guilty to criminal charges related to paying more than $20 million in kickbacks and bribing a state Sen. to preserve a loophole in state law that enabled him to charge insurers high prices for spinal hardware which amounted up to $160,000 for the screws, rods and cages implanted in one person's back.

Health care consumers need to identify these health care fraudsters and report them to attempt to salvage the health care system. People need to remember that he/she could receive a monetary reward for being a whistle blower.

Whistle blowers are people who expose unethical or illegal wrongdoing within companies by reporting it internally to superiors or externally to the media, government authorities, or specialized attorneys. They can be either current or past employees (insiders), or outside individuals who are familiar with the unlawful conduct, and are not required to be U.S. citizens. If you properly report Medicare fraud, you may be entitled to a significant whistleblower reward.

40. Obstetrics Gynecology Fraud

Obstetrics & Gynecology is the medical specialty that deals with obstetrics and gynecology. Postgraduate training programs for both aspects are usually combined, preparing the practicing obstetrician-gynecologist to be adept at the care of female reproductive organs' health and at the management of pregnancy, although many doctors go on to develop subspecialty interests in one field or the other.

A doctor from Michigan was convicted of one count of conspiracy to commit health care fraud after a jury trial lasting approximately two weeks. He was a physician for a home visiting physician service based in Chicago, from 2012 to 2013. The evidence at trial showed that the doctor visited patients who did not qualify for visiting physician services, and these visits were then billed to Medicare at the highest billing codes. For example, the evidence showed that the doctor billed Medicare for home visits that required complex, 40 or 60 minute examinations, but would instead rush through as many as 22 home visits per day, averaging about 15 minutes or less with each patient, so he could make more money. The evidence also showed that he ordered unnecessary tests, in order to receive larger bonuses.

As part of their guilty pleas, two obstetricians admitted to seeing patients who did not need their services and for whom bills were submitted to Medicare at the highest billing codes. In connection with this case, each pleaded guilty to one count of conspiracy to commit health care fraud in March 2017 and December 2016, respectively.

In another case Lake MI Mobile Doctors billed Medicare approximately $17.1 million as a result of the scheme in which these doctors participated. The evidence showed. The FBI and HHS–OIG investigated the case, which was brought as part of the Medicare Fraud Strike Force under the supervision of the Criminal Division's Fraud Section and the US Attorney's Office for the Eastern District of Michigan.

The Fraud Section leads the Medicare Fraud Strike Force. Since its inception in March 2007, the Medicare Fraud Strike Force, now operating in nine cities across the country, has charged nearly 3,000 defendants who have collectively billed the Medicare program for more than $11 billion. In addition, the HHS Centers for Medicare & Medicaid Services, working in conjunction with the HHS–OIG, are taking steps to increase accountability and decrease the presence of fraudulent providers.

Another doctor pleaded guilty in 2009 to insurance fraud and was ordered to repay $38,000. He now faces disciplinary actions ranging from a public reprimand, probation or revoked medical license. The doctor began using birth control devices made in Mexico in 2004. The Mexican devices cost approximately $30 each, but documents show that the doctor billed Medi-Cal for 10 times that much. Over two years, the doctor inserted about 110 Mexican IUDs into patients and received approximately $38,000 in Medi-Cal payments.

A gynecologist from Monroe, N.C., has agreed to pay $750,000 to settle allegations that she billed state Medicaid for six years' worth of services never rendered. This doctor owns an obstetrics and gynecology practice. The civil settlement was reached after a probe of her billing practices found false claims for 1,009 patients from 2003 to 2008. The $750,000 settlement is double the amount of billings in question.

An obstetrics/gynecology physician was suspended from a hospital for disruptive behavior and also prescribed anxiety and weight loss drugs without proper paperwork, the Iowa Board of Medicine claims. An obstetrician of Port Byron, Ill, is charged with incompetency, unethical conduct, fraud, and deception and engaging in a practice that is harmful or detrimental to the public. The medical board may revoke his medical license if it rules that his conduct poses an "immediate threat to the public or his patients.

He provided prenatal care from February 2011 to the present without properly informing patients that he did not have hospital delivery privileges, the board charges. In early 2012, he failed to manage a patient's preeclampsia, failed to perform fetal well-being studies and failed to make appropriate arrangements for delivery of the baby, the board charges. He also prescribed excessive doses of Xanax a potentially addictive anxiety drug to at least two patients and phentermine to patients for weight loss without appropriate documentation, the board charges.

The doctor was charged on six felony counts, including one count of unlawful acts concerning computers, one count of making false claims to the Medicaid program and four counts of obstruction of a Medicaid fraud investigation. He was judged guilty by Leavenworth

County District Court Judge Gunnar A. Sundby after he pled no contest. The crimes occurred between Jan. 2009 and Dec. 2013 and included billing Medicaid for services he did not perform and altering patient records.

A Louisiana woman underwent a hysterectomy in 2007, performed by her longtime gynecologist. Her bladder was injured during the surgery, and a urologist was called to repair the injury. The patient sued the gynecologist, alleging negligence in injuring the bladder. The patient claimed that the physician had suffered a serious injury in a fall in 2004 that affected his dexterity, and that he never informed her of the extent of his injury and risks associated with it.

The physician maintained that the bladder injury was a risk of the surgery about which the patient had been advised, and it was recognized and repaired appropriately. A motion for summary judgment was granted for the physician on this claim. He argued that his injury affected only his ability to stand in surgery all day.

According to information presented in court, an obstetrician/gynecologist, formerly practiced in Beaumont, Texas, was enrolled as a Texas Medicaid Provider. As part of his practice, he commonly submitted claims for ultrasounds and microbial identification tests, but as he was aware, his office was not capable of performing the tests. At the end of February 2005, two physicians practicing with this doctor left the practice and took the ultrasound and microbial testing equipment with them.

From March 2005 until August 2005, the doctor did not have access to ultrasound equipment, and from March 2005 until November 2005, he did not have access to microbial testing equipment. However, during these times, the doctor continued to bill Medicaid for both tests and submitted claims for hundreds of unperformed tests resulting in the fraudulent payment of $76,683 from the Texas Medicaid program.

An obstetrics and gynecology physician was arrested for allegedly defrauding the Florida Medicaid program and prescribing medically unnecessary controlled substances to pregnant patients. According to the investigation, the owner of a medical practice, performed and submitted claims for medically unnecessary procedures and billed for services not rendered. This doctor also allegedly prescribed medically unnecessary controlled substances to pregnant women by means of written orders or prescriptions.

The 50-year-old individual is facing felony charges for posing as a doctor and offering unsuspecting patients free gynecological services. After busting this doctor in an undercover sting, investigators are now trying to identify Dallas women who may have been victimized by this doctor who advertised his services which included pap smears and "vaginal irrigation" in a weekly newspaper.

This individual ran his scam, remarkably, from an office at a self-storage facility, where he greeted one female undercover agent wearing white pants and a "white medical scrub shirt," according to Dallas County Sheriff's Department reports. He completed the look by wearing a stethoscope around his neck. This individual was being held without bond in a Dallas lockup, faces a maximum of ten years in prison if convicted of the medical charade.

A warrant has been issued for the arrest of a 68-year-old obstetrician on five counts of video voyeurism after a patient accused the doctor of photographing her private parts during a routine exam. The doctor snapped pictures of the patient's "pubic region and buttocks" without her consent on April 1, 2014.

Arkansas State Police issued a warrant to seize the doctor's cell phone on April 10. According to the warrant, "found in the deleted images within the hard-drive of the cellular telephone were numerous images of nude females that appear to have been taken in a medical office during medical examinations." Also recovered during the examination were what appear to be photographs of the woman who first reported the crime.

According to the evidence presented during the one-week trial, another obstetrician joined a conspiracy to bill Medicare for medically unnecessary neurological tests some of which involved sending an electrical current through the arms and legs of the patients. According to court documents, clinic employees, who lacked any meaningful training, administered the diagnostic tests, and the patients never received any follow-up treatment by neurologists.

Evidence at trial showed that the patients were not referred to the clinics by their primary care physicians, or for any other legitimate purpose, but rather were recruited with prescriptions for controlled substances, cash payments, and fast food. The three clinics then billed the Medicare program for various diagnostic tests that were medically unnecessary. This doctor exposed patients to electrical currents for neurological testing solely to generate money for himself at the expense of the Medicare program. In each case, the delivery was actually performed by clinic staff doctors, who the doctor knew did not submit bills to Medicaid,

The doctor's former girlfriend, pleaded guilty to obstructing justice by helping the doctor falsify billing records. She testified the doctor would go to a medical center office, where he practiced, and find a patient on Medicaid who delivered a baby at the hands of the hospital staff doctors. The doctor then extracted sufficient medical information from the records to submit fraudulent bills to the Medicaid program alleging that he had delivered the babies, prosecutors said. The doctor once billed for a single delivery when the mother actually had delivered twins, In another billing, he asserted he had performed a vaginal delivery on behalf of a woman who had undergone a Caesarean section.

Health care consumers need to identify these health care fraudsters and report them to attempt to salvage the health care system. People need to remember that he/she could receive a monetary reward for being a whistle blower.

Whistle blowers are people who expose unethical or illegal wrongdoing within companies by reporting it internally to superiors or externally to the media, government authorities, or specialized attorneys. They can be either current or past employees (insiders), or outside individuals who are familiar with the unlawful conduct, and are not required to be U.S. citizens. If you properly report Medicare fraud, you may be entitled to a significant whistleblower reward.

41. Oncology Fraud

Oncology is a branch of medicine that deals with the prevention, diagnosis and treatment of cancer. A medical professional who practices oncology is an oncologist. The name's etymological origin is the Greek word meaning tumor,

The three components which have improved survival in cancer are: 1. Prevention by reduction of risk factors like tobacco and alcohol consumption. 2. Early diagnosis with screening of common cancers and comprehensive diagnosis and staging of the cancer. 3. Treatment by multimodality management by discussion in tumor board and treatment in a comprehensive cancer center. Treating cancer is a $200 billion a year business.

All cancers are different, and no one treatment works for every cancer or everybody. Even two people with the same diagnosis may need different treatments. Scammers take advantage of the feelings that can accompany a diagnosis of cancer. They promote unproven and potentially dangerous remedies like black salve, essiac tea, or laetrile with claims that the products are both "natural" and effective. But "natural" doesn't mean either safe or effective when it comes to using these treatments for cancer. In fact, a product that is labeled "natural," can be more than ineffective: it can be downright harmful. The National Cancer Institute states that the medical costs of cancer care are $125 billion, with a projected 39 percent increase to $173 billion by 2020.

A former "pharmaceutical designer and consultant" was charged with illegally practicing medicine after he was caught dispensing expired pharmaceuticals and bags of dirt as "treatment" to patients dying of cancer. This individual age 69, reportedly charged a female cancer patient $2,000 for a satchel containing literal garbage, including several plastic bags filled with soil, empty capsules, expired drugs and other random materials.

This individual isn't a doctor, and he never received any formal education beyond high school. Most oncologists don't make their money by treating patients, but by selling cancer drugs. In fact, according to the Journal of the American Medical Association, as much as 75% of the average oncologist's earnings come from selling chemotherapy drugs in his or her office and at a substantially marked-up price.

Pharmaceutical companies not only hire charismatic people to charm doctors, exaggerate drug benefits and underplay side effects, but they also pay oncologists kickbacks to push their drugs. For example, AstraZeneca, Inc. had to pay $280 million in civil penalties and $63 million in criminal penalties to the federal government after it paid kickbacks to doctors for promoting its prostate cancer drug. In a rare joint action with attorneys general for each of the 50 states, the Federal Trade Commission says four cancer charities run by extended members of the same family conned donors out of $187 million from 2008 through 2012 and spent almost nothing to help actual cancer patients.

An oncologist, who owns hematology oncology centers, is accused of giving unnecessary chemotherapy to patients who didn't need it and diagnosing cancer when it wasn't apparent. According to the complaint, the oncologist defrauded federally funded Medicare out of about $35 million over a two-year period. Prosecutors said syringes were re-used and different patients' chemotherapy drugs were drawn from the same bag at Rose Cancer Center.

A Florida based oncology practice, which has offices in Florida has agreed to pay nearly $34.7 million to the United States government to settle a Medicare fraud lawsuit claiming it performed and billed for radiation procedures that were not medically necessary. The lawsuit was brought against the nation's leading provider of cancer care services by a whistle-blower, a former physicist at the practice. The settlement relates to the use of a medical procedure called the Gamma function used to measure the exit dose radiating from a patient after the patient receives radiation treatment. The practice, knowingly and improperly billed for this procedure under circumstances where the procedure served no medically appropriate purpose. This practice in some instances performed tests that were not only medically unnecessary, but that no one had been trained to properly interpret, thereby allegedly causing the taxpayers to pay for useless tests.

The dispute involved the training protocols of certain staff in the utilization of GAMMA, and was limited to its early implementation and startup activities at new facility locations across the country, the statement said. The company implemented GAMMA across all centers to ensure every patient had access to this technology. The GAMMA function was described as a state-of-the art radiation dose calculation system developed, implemented by these physicians to optimize patient outcomes.

Another settlement announced resolves allegations that an oncology practice submitted claims to Medicare and Tricare for fluorescence in situ hybridization, or "FISH," tests that were not medically necessary. FISH tests are laboratory tests performed on urine that can detect genetic abnormalities associated with bladder cancer.

A Texas teenager who claimed to be dying of cancer was arrested after investigators found that she lied in order to receive donations. The teenager, 19, was indicted April 19 on a state felony charge of theft of property of $1,500 to $20,000, according to court documents. She allegedly received $17,000 in donations and gifts. She claimed that she had cancer began in January 2011. She told classmates at a high school that doctors had given her six months to live. She claimed to suffer from leukemia as a child in Kansas City and that it had returned.

Many medical conditions involve incredibly expensive diagnosis and treatment and much of that expense is in the form of profits paid to the doctors performing the diagnosing and treating. In many cases, those profits reach to the millions of dollars. Insurance fraud, Medicare fraud, Medicaid fraud, and a medical billing system that hides the true costs of medical care from patients all conspire to attract the greedy and unscrupulous.

There were subscriptions to dating websites, meals at Hooters and purchases at Victoria's Secret not to mention Jet Ski joy rides and couples' cruises to the Caribbean. All of it was paid for with the nearly $200 million donated to cancer charities, and was enjoyed by the healthy friends and family members of those running the groups, in what government officials said Tuesday was one of the largest charity fraud cases ever.

Federal authorities are investigating whether one of the region's largest and most prominent providers of cancer care, defrauded taxpayers out of millions of dollars a year. A whistle blower's complaint accuses the organization of billing for more expensive procedures than were actually performed, billing for procedures that never were performed and performing medically unnecessary procedures on patients, among other violations, according to the source.

The lengthy list of allegations against another oncology practice includes: Employees knowingly submitted false records to Medicare and Medicaid, in an arrangement that placed profits over patients. At times, no physician was present to directly supervise radiation and diagnostic scans, in violation of Medicare guidelines. The staffers offered numerous unnecessary treatments and services to patients. The staffers recruited and treated patients who have terminal cancer and are recommended for hospice care, where further radiation treatment is harmful or ineffective. The patients are treated, not because of a diagnosis that the cancer can be treated, but instead to bill Medicare and the other insurance programs. Staff, furthermore, re-treated areas on patients who have already been treated with radiation, in excess of prescribed dosage limits, again to make as much money as possible and at the expense of patient safety.

The practice demanded payment for services it hasn't performed, such as weekly treatment management sessions that require physicians to meet with their patients, examine them and go over their records with them. The whistle blower alleged the reviews often didn't take place. Another treatment that didn't always take place was an imaging guided radiation therapy, or IGRT, scan that was supposed to take place before every treatment. The physicians allowed registered nurses to fill out prescriptions for medications. The practice also regularly offered "kickbacks" to patients by waiving their co-pays for the treatments the practice was provided to them.

Another oncology practice physician was sentenced to pay a $500,000 fine, forfeit $1.2 million, and make restitution to Medicare in the amount of $1.7 million for purchasing unapproved foreign cancer drugs and billing Medicare as if the drugs were legitimate. In pleading guilty, the practice admitted that it had purchased $3.4 million of foreign cancer drugs, knowing they had not been approved by the U.S. Food and Drug Administration for use in the United States.

From 2007 to 2011, this office purchased these drugs for significantly less than market value in the U.S. and then submitted claims to Medicare at the full reimbursement price. To conceal the scheme, the office fraudulently used Medicare reimbursement codes for approved cancer drugs, as Medicare does not pay for unapproved drugs.

In another case, providers engaged in a billing fraud scheme from 2007 through 2011 which included billing for radiation oncology services that were not supervised by a physician as required by Medicare, Medicaid and TRICARE. Although physician supervision was a requirement for reimbursement, the defendant providers, nonetheless, billed for services when the physicians were on vacation and otherwise not on site. In addition, the defendant providers billed for services that were never performed, an illegal practice known as "phantom billing." They also billed the government twice for services that were only performed once, a fraudulent practice known as "double-billing."

A Florida oncologist was charged with giving cancer patients medications, including chemotherapy drugs, from other countries that were not approved by the federal Food and Drug Administration. The oncologist and her staff gave patients cheaper, misbranded drugs that weren't registered or approved for use in the United States. She then billed the taxpayer-funded Medicare program and private insurance companies for the illegal prescriptions, claiming that she was actually using the FDA-approved versions. The oncologist pocketed the extra money, according to the indictment.

Law enforcement officials arrested a man in Northern California who was practicing medicine without a license at a fake oncology center. For more than five years, this individual has been treating cancer patients out of an office in California. He operated a clinic that offered alternative cancer therapies for patients with late-stage forms of the disease who had run out of effective treatment options. A 49-year-old female patient reported him to officials. The woman says he gave her fake medicine in powder and liquid form, expired drugs, bags of dirt and a bill for $2,000.

The cancer industry is probably the most prosperous business in the United States. In 2014, there were an estimated 1,665,540 new cancer cases diagnosed and 585,720 cancer deaths in the US. $6 billion of tax-payer funds are cycled through various federal agencies for cancer research, such as the National Cancer Institute (NCI). The NCI states that the medical costs of cancer care are $125 billion, with a projected 39 percent increase to $173 billion by 2020.

The owners of a Kentucky cancer clinic have paid $3.7 million to settle claims that they extended the period of chemotherapy for their patients. The clinic submitted false claims for payment to the Medicare, Medicaid and the military's medical provider for extending the duration of chemotherapy infusion treatment to patients and inappropriately billing office visits for infusion therapy. The settlement agreement says that the physicians from 2006 to 2013 unnecessarily and improperly extended the duration of chemotherapy infusion treatment times for their patients, so they could make more money. It also says they and their clinic falsely billed for office evaluations of patients receiving chemotherapy. The oncologists in question gave patients the appropriate dose of chemotherapy, but diluted it and prolonged treatment for hours so that they could bill more to Medicaid and Medicare, which pay in part based on how long a procedure takes.

Furthermore, a prominent Orange County cancer doctor has agreed to plead guilty to charges of defrauding Medicare and other insurers of up to $1 million for injectable cancer medications that never were provided. Rather than give a diluted substance, this doctor gave nothing to patients. Health care consumers need to identify these health care fraudsters and report them to attempt to salvage the health care system. People need to remember that he/she could receive a monetary reward for being a whistle blower.

Whistle blowers are people who expose unethical or illegal wrongdoing within companies by reporting it internally to superiors or externally to the media, government authorities, or specialized attorneys. They can be either current or past employees (insiders), or outside individuals who are familiar with the unlawful conduct, and are not required to be U.S. citizens. If you properly report Medicare fraud, you may be entitled to a significant whistleblower reward.

42. Ophthalmology Fraud

Ophthalmology is the branch of medicine that deals with the anatomy, physiology and diseases of the eyeball and orbit. An ophthalmologist is a specialist in medical and surgical eye problems. Their credentials include an M.D. or D.O. degree, and an additional four years of residency. Ophthalmologists are allowed to medically treat eye disease, implement laser therapy, and perform incisional surgery when warranted.

In the summer of 2009, a prominent Indiana ophthalmologist and his wife were accused in a U.S. District Court of medical fraud and days later, died in a reported murder-suicide. The couple was accused of making false and fraudulent cataract diagnoses and performing unnecessary cataract surgeries. Less than a week after facing charges, the two were found dead of gunshot wounds in their office. He reportedly died of a self-inflicted gunshot to the head, and his wife died of multiple wounds to the chest.

Their health care fraud scheme involved three false and fraudulent components: billings for medically unnecessary tests, up-coded billings, and double billings. To increase income, they that many patients receive a battery of diagnostic tests, many of which were not medical necessary. Claims for these medically unnecessary tests were submitted to Medicare and private insurers for reimbursement.

The ophthalmologist also engaged in a practice of up-coding certain tests by claiming his practice was entitled to a higher than warranted reimbursement rate. Finally, this practice was supposed to be paid one amount for tests performed on both eyes, but it fraudulently submitted bills to health insurance plans that resulted in this practice being paid twice, once for each eye. The government alleges the loss attributable to the health care fraud scheme is $1,702,567.89.

An ophthalmologist was indicted in June by a federal grand jury for multiple counts of health care fraud, wire fraud and criminal conspiracy. He was charged with billing Medicare, Medicaid and private insurance carriers for unnecessary cataract procedures. He had offices in Indiana, and his wife was employed as the office manager in the practice.

Another case involved the chairperson of a university opthalmalology department. Between 1996 and 2007, he caused thousands of false claims to be submitted to health care benefit programs with false charges totaling more than $4.5 million for services rendered to patients whom he did not personally see or evaluate. At his direction, Ophthalmology Department staff employees would stack patient charts outside his office door at the main campus of the University Hospital. The patients had been seen by other physicians in the office, but he falsified the charts by making notations indicating that he had personally seen and evaluated the patients. In fact, this doctor was outside of the state in other locations on some of the days that he claimed to have treated patients, including Las Vegas, Nevada; Sarasota, Florida; and Indian Wells, California.

He also signed the patient charts and filled out fee slips for the services that he falsely claimed to have provided. As a result, health care benefits programs, including Medicare and private health insurers, made payments on fraudulent claims in excess of $1.8 million. This doctor also made false statements in the medical records of patients attesting that he had personally seen the patients, when he knew; he had created these false records solely for the purpose of submitting fraudulent billings to health care benefit programs.

A federal judge has ordered an Orlando, Fla.; ophthalmologist held without bail on charges he defrauded Medicare of $7 million, according to published reports. This ophthalmologist is alleged to have falsely diagnosed hundreds of patients with macular degeneration and imminent blindness, then performed sham laser surgeries and unnecessary follow-up care before billing Medicare and commercial insurers for the services from the mid-2000s to 2011.

According to a federal grand jury's indictment, which charged the 56-year-old physician with 20 counts of Medicare fraud on April 24, this doctor used a low-power laser that had no impact on patients' vision. This doctor a Florida ophthalmologist with offices in Leesburg and West Orange County, was accused of bilking Medicare out of $7 million by allegedly lying to his patients, providing unnecessary and phony surgery to correct nonexistent problems, and then billing Medicare for the phantom treatment. Federal agents report that this doctor billed Medicare for $72 million over the past decade. The insurer suspended his certification last year after the state began investigating three medical-malpractice complaints filed against him.

On April 24, a federal jury in Jacksonville indicted the 56-year-old on 20 counts of healthcare fraud. This doctor pleaded not guilty in one of the largest ophthalmology Medicare fraud cases in Florida. Throughout the scheme, which occurred from 2006 to 2011, he convinced many of his patients that they needed to be treated for wet macular degeneration to prevent blindness. The chronic eye disease causes vision loss due to abnormal blood vessels leaking fluid or blood into the eye.

According to the complaint, another ophthalmologist frequently visited area nursing homes and often claimed to treat more than 100 nursing-home patients in a single day. The complaint alleges that on certain dates, these services would have required more than 20 hours' worth of direct patient care per day, and that this doctor was not working inside these nursing homes more than 8 hours per day.

The complaint also claims that the defendants sought payment for routine monthly eye examinations that were unreasonable and unnecessary given the patients' conditions. Many nursing-home patients received an eye examination from this ophthalmologist every four to five weeks for five years or more. At times, he billed Medicare for certain eye examinations more than any other eye doctor in the United States.

In another case, the complaint accuses the defendants of violating the False Claims Act. If found liable, the defendants would face financial penalties between $5,500 and $11,000 per false claim, and would have to repay Medicare and Medicaid three times the amount of the U.S. Government's loss for the fraud.

Under the guise of caring for nursing-home residents, several eye doctors misused the Medicare and Medicaid programs. Individuals paying for eye care with money from their own pocket would not be expected to pay a doctor to simply monitor their vision with a monthly exam, especially if the exams were as brief and superficial as what the eye doctor provided. Health care programs funded with taxpayer dollars are no different."

Charges centered on an ophthalmologist's use of a highly controversial and unapproved laser procedure. This doctor has already had to repay Medicare $8.9 million and has been asked to return another $32 million. National health regulators and federal judges agreed he wasn't entitled to the $57.3 million he made by using a single vial of ranibizumab injection (Lucentis, Genentech) for treatment of wet age-related macular degeneration on multiple patients. The practice is known as multi-dosing.

Additional charges centered on the doctor's use of a highly controversial and unapproved laser procedure. In addition, since the treatment is not approved and there was no billing code for it. The doctor was billing Medicare using the wrong billing code which is reserved for laser photocoagulation of a choroidal lesion. This code is rarely used since the advent of intraocular injections.

The U.S. government has sued a North Hollywood ophthalmologist convicted of submitting fraudulent Medicare claims in an effort to recover at least $150,000. The ophthalmologist was found guilty last year in Los Angeles Superior Court in Van Nuys of 36 grand theft counts in connection with the bogus billings for eye surgeries that never occurred. The doctor was sentenced to 16 months in state prison and was fined $686,000.

A physician affiliated in the early 1990s with a Doctors Hospital and Eye Center pleaded guilty Friday to a federal fraud charge and agreed to cooperate in a continuing federal investigation.

This doctor pleaded guilty to ordering hundreds of unnecessary tests for patients undergoing cataract surgery and admitting hundreds of others to his Hospital under false pretenses. In his plea agreement with authorities, he admitted pocketing $11,300 in payoffs from one undisclosed eye care official for ordering hundreds of unnecessary allergy tests in 1992 and 1993. This doctor admitted he cleared patients for surgery before testing them properly. For nearly a year in 1993 and 1994, he said he admitted about 100 patients a month to the hospital that didn't need to be hospitalized.

An ophthalmology office manager and son of the ophthalmologist pleaded guilty last summer to committing health care fraud by submitting false bills to public and private health benefit programs and conspiring to defraud the United States through a family scheme to evade paying federal income taxes. He's agreed to pay $2.5 million in restitution.

He and his late father ran an ophthalmology practice. They required patients to undergo unnecessary testing, double-billed patients for certain tests and then put the revenue in a bank account of a shell.

The father and son used about $3 million in funds to start building a multimillion-dollar 35,000-square-foot-house, complete with a helipad and tennis pavilion, for Anthony Neal and his wife. It was to be linked through a heated tunnel to Dr. Neal's house 75 yards away, where the younger Neal and his wife lived in the basement. The house was never finished. The father and son concealed from the IRS more than $1.3 million in company revenue each year from 2009 to 2013.

Health care consumers need to identify these health care fraudsters and report them to attempt to salvage the health care system. People need to remember that he/she could receive a monetary reward for being a whistle blower.

Whistle blowers are people who expose unethical or illegal wrongdoing within companies by reporting it internally to superiors or externally to the media, government authorities, or specialized attorneys. They can be either current or past employees (insiders), or outside individuals who are familiar with the unlawful conduct, and are not required to be U.S. citizens. If you properly report Medicare fraud, you may be entitled to a significant whistleblower reward.

43. Orthopedic Surgery Fraud

Orthopedic surgery or orthopedics is the branch of surgery concerned with conditions involving the musculoskeletal system. Orthopedic surgeons use both surgical and nonsurgical means to treat musculoskeletal trauma, spine diseases, sports injuries, degenerative diseases, infections, tumors, and congenital disorders

An orthopedic surgeon accused of botching or faking hundreds of surgeries surrendered to authorities and was charged with one count of healthcare fraud. The charges state that from 2007 through 2011. A doctor reported performing thousands of surgical procedures, often as many as 20 or more in a single day, included many which were never really carried out. This and the medical group submitted claims in excess of $35 million to health care providers. The federal government claims that as part of his scheme to defraud insurance providers, he routinely saw up to 90 patients in a single office day, charging insurance carriers an additional $3.5 million in claims during that time period.

Another orthopedic surgeon was charged as the ringleader in one of the state's biggest health fraud schemes, which included unnecessary operations by an untrained assistant that scarred patients forever, according to indictments unsealed Tuesday.

Another physician defrauded insurance companies out of $150 million. Nearly two dozen patients were told that this doctor would perform surgery on them, only to have his physician's assistant who had not attended medical school operate once they were under anesthesia. The doctor wasn't even present for the surgeries. All 21 patients sustained lasting scars and many required additional surgeries and suffered physical and psychological trauma as a result of their experience in this clinic. While performing surgeries at University of Cincinnati Health and West Chester (Ohio) Hospital between 2010 and 2013, a spine surgeon submitted more than $7 million in Medicare reimbursements. A federal grand jury indicted the spine surgeon for healthcare fraud and performing unnecessary surgeries.

The United States specifically alleged that nine hospitals overcharged Medicare between 2000 and 2008 when performing kyphoplasty, a minimally-invasive procedure used to treat certain spinal fractures that often are due to osteoporosis. In many cases, the procedure can be performed safely as a less costly out-patient procedure, but the government contends that the hospitals performed the procedure on an in-patient basis in order to increase their Medicare billings.

The settlement with these facilities follows the settlements that the government reached in May and September 2009 with nine other hospitals for alleged kyphoplasty-related Medicare fraud claims, as well as the government's May 2008 settlement with Medtronic Spine LLC, corporate successor to Kyphon Inc. Medtronic Spine paid $75 million to settle allegations that the company defrauded Medicare by counseling hospital providers to perform kyphoplasty procedures as an in-patient procedure, even though in many cases the minimally-invasive procedure should have been done on an out-patient basis.

Five Modesto doctors are among more than two dozen physicians, pharmacists, business owners and a physician assistant charged in a $40 million fraudulent medical billing and kickback scheme, authorities announced Thursday. Authorities allege the scam took place from 2011 to 2015 and involved more than 13,000 patients. Authorities said $40 million was billed to insurance companies, and the defendants were paid about $23.2 million.

The United States contends that it has certain civil claims a group of orthopedic specialists arising from the medical group billing federal health care programs for services that were not medically necessary and reasonable. Specifically, this group sought reimbursement for millions of dollars' of health care claims that were questionable. This group knowingly billed for certain claims as "incident to" physician supervision when no physician was present or there was no verification of any physician being present.

This group knowingly scheduled patients' follow-up operative visits from 12 weeks following surgery to 14 weeks in an effort to bill for a separate visit outside the normal Medicare 90 days Diagnosis-Related Group charge. The group knowingly used and billed for ultrasound-guided injections routinely even in the absence of medical necessity; and knowingly billed for certain physical therapy claims using Modifier KX so as to exceed the Medicare cap on physical therapy, despite the absence of medical necessity.

Visco supplements, such as Synvisc and Orthovisc, are injections approved by the Food and Drug Administration for the treatment of osteoarthritis pain in the knee. Visco supplements are reimbursed by Medicare, Medicaid, and other federal health care programs at a set rate based on the average sales price of the domestic product. The government contended that a clinic knowingly purchased deeply discounted viscosupplements that were reimported from foreign countries and billed them to state and federal health care programs in order to profit from the reimbursement system, when such reimported visco supplements were not reimbursable by those programs. Allegedly, the reimported product included labeling in foreign languages and in English for additional uses not approved in the United States, which demonstrated that the product was reimported. Moreover, because the product was reimported, the government alleged there was no manufacturer assurance that it had not been tampered with or that it was stored appropriately.

Fifteen individuals associated with an orthopedic surgery practice in Los Angeles have been indicted for participating in illegal patient referrals, faked medical evaluations that led to unnecessary procedures, botched surgeries performed by people who weren't trained to perform surgery, and, almost as an afterthought, Medicare fraud. The Medical Board of California put the orthopedic surgeon on probation in 2010 for letting his physician's assistant perform surgeries and canceled his license in 2013; he's believed to have fled the country after Park was arrested on murder charges and may or may not have just been arrested in Germany.

The schemes involved tens of millions of dollars in illegal kickbacks to dozens of doctors, chiropractors and others. As a result of the illegal payments, thousands of patients were referred to Pacific Hospital in Long Beach, where they underwent spinal surgeries that led to more than $580 million in bills being fraudulently submitted during the last eight years of the scheme alone. Many of the fraudulent claims were paid by the California worker's compensation system and the federal government. In a second, similar scheme that also involved spinal surgeries, doctors received illegal kickbacks for referrals to a Hawaiian Gardens hospital.

In a series of related cases announced today, the former chief financial officer of a Long Beach, California, hospital, two orthopedic surgeons and two others have been charged in long-running health care fraud schemes that illegally referred thousands of patients for spinal surgeries and generated nearly $600 million in fraudulent billings over an eight-year period. Two of the defendants have pleaded guilty and three others have agreed to plead guilty in the coming weeks. All five defendants have agreed to cooperate in the government's ongoing investigation into kickbacks for patient referrals and fraudulent bills for spinal surgeries.

The schemes involved tens of millions of dollars in illegal kickbacks to dozens of doctors, chiropractors and others. As a result of the illegal payments, thousands of patients were referred to Pacific Hospital in Long Beach, where they underwent spinal surgeries that led to more than $580 million in bills being fraudulently submitted during the last eight years of the scheme alone. Many of the fraudulent claims were paid by the California worker's compensation system and the federal government.

An orthopedic surgeon of San Pedro, California, the former CFO of Pacific Hospital in Long Beach, who pleaded guilty on Sept. 4 to a criminal information charging him with participating in a conspiracy that engaged in mail fraud, honest services fraud, money laundering, paying or receiving kickbacks in connection with a federal health care program and violating the Travel Act, specifically, interstate travel in aid of a racketeering enterprise.

A chiropractor who formerly resided in San Juan Capistrano, California, and owned several businesses based in Costa Mesa, California, was charged today in a criminal information that alleges one count of conspiracy to commit mail fraud, honest services fraud, money laundering and violations of the Travel Act. In a plea agreement also filed today, Ivar admitted that for well over a decade, he had an agreement with the owner of Pacific Hospital to refer patients in exchange for a monthly retainer. The surgeon, who admitted recruiting chiropractors and doctors to refer patients to Tri-City in exchange for kickbacks, was scheduled to be sentenced on April 8, 2016.

An orthopedic surgeon was charged last week with filing a false tax return. The doctor admitted in a plea agreement that he failed to report income received from kickback payments and is expected to be arraigned next month.

All five defendants have agreed to cooperate with the government's ongoing investigation, dubbed "Operation Spinal Cap," into the kickback schemes, which involved dozens of surgeons, orthopedic specialists, chiropractors, marketers and other medical professionals. All of the defendants will be required to pay restitution to the victims of the scheme, which in one case will be at least $20 million.

The owner and CEO of a hospital in Long Beach until late 2013, ran a 15-year-long scheme in which he and others billed workers' compensation insurers and the U.S. Department of Labor hundreds of millions of dollars for spinal surgeries and other procedures performed on patients who had been referred by dozens of doctors, chiropractors and others who were paid illegal kickbacks.

As part of the scheme, the conspirators typically paid a kickback of $15,000 for each lumbar fusion surgery and $10,000 for each cervical fusion surgery. Some of the patients lived hundreds of miles away from Pacific Hospital and closer to other qualified medical facilities. The patients were not informed that medical professionals had been offered kickbacks to induce them to refer the surgeries to Pacific Hospital. From 2005 through 2013, only part of the overall scheme, the hospital billed insurers more than $580 million for spinal surgeries on more than 4,400 patients. Insurers paid the hospital more than $226 million for the surgeries performed as a result of illegal kickbacks. Injured workers were treated like livestock by doctors and hospitals that paid or accepted kickbacks and bribes in exchange for referrals. Injured workers are put at risk when their medical treatment is based on kickbacks and bribes instead of their medical needs.

The surgeries at a hospital involved use of spinal surgery hardware that was distributed to a hospital at inflated prices through his company. Using proceeds from the sale of the hardware, a doctor paid a 5 percent kickback to Tri-City and kickbacks of up to $20,000 per surgery to the doctors and chiropractors who referred the patients. In addition, kickbacks were made to doctors in return for referrals of patients for toxicology tests though a separate company, Platinum Medical. The scheme resulted in several million dollars in losses to insurers.

An orthopedic surgeon who previously worked at the Walter Reed Army Medical Center in Washington, had been accused by four former colleagues there of falsifying research on a bone-growth product made by Medtronic that was used on severely injured soldiers. He was also accused of forging the other doctors' signatures when he submitted a research report to a medical journal last year.

The surgeon has been a consultant to Medtronic. The company has also paid for some of his research and writings. Medtronic, the nation's largest medical-device maker, announced Wednesday that it was suspending the doctor's consulting contract, which started in August 2006 as he left Walter Reed for the university position. Medtronic has declined to provide details of its consulting payments but said it had no involvement with the disputed research. Army investigators said the doctor's study had cast Infuse, a bioengineered bone-growth product sold by Medtronic, in a misleadingly favorable light compared with conventional bone grafts in repairing severely shattered shin bones of American soldiers injured in the Iraq war.

Recently a disturbing article was previously found in Business Week, concerning the growth of a facility in Tampa known as Laser Spine Institute. Specifically, the article discusses the rapid growth of this facility which focuses on offering outpatient laser spine surgery as basically a cookie cutter solution to most disco genic spine pathology and symptomatology. Unfortunately, many of these surgeries have turned out to be unwarranted and have proven to be unsuccessful.

Insurance carriers have strongly scrutinized laser spine procedures and are reluctant to settle such claims as they see such procedures as unwarranted and based on questionable science. Bloomberg News' David Armstrong reported that the booming business at for-profit outpatient laser surgery clinics comes at a high price for insurers and some patients. Furthermore, the rate of serious complaints is higher than those for other outpatient procedures.

Health care consumers need to identify these health care fraudsters and report them to attempt to salvage the health care system. People need to remember that he/she could receive a monetary reward for being a whistle blower.

Whistle blowers are people who expose unethical or illegal wrongdoing within companies by reporting it internally to superiors or externally to the media, government authorities, or specialized attorneys. They can be either current or past employees (insiders), or outside individuals who are familiar with the unlawful conduct, and are not required to be U.S. citizens. If you properly report Medicare fraud, you may be entitled to a significant whistleblower reward.

44. Otolaryngology Fraud

Otolaryngology (ENT) is a branch of medicine that focuses on the ears, nose and throat (ENT), and sinuses. Otolaryngologists (ENT doctors) diagnose and treat problems with the ears, nose, throat, and sinuses. Problems may include hearing loss, throat infections, sinusitis (sinus infection) and problems with the nose, such as a nasal polyp (growth in the nose).

Between August 2004 and September 2010, an ENT specialist was the owner and operator of a medical treatment otolaryngology facility. This doctor treated a patient with the initials J.F. for nasal problems and billed Blue Cross Blue Shield for the services he purportedly performed.The doctor admitted he filed fraudulent claims with Blue Cross Blue Shield for medical procedures that were not performed during office visits. This doctor submitted claims for approximately 900 nasal endoscopies he purportedly conducted on the patient, when only a few were actually performed.

He also admitted he filed fraudulent claims for office visits and medical procedures that purportedly occurred while he was away on vacation. Between September 6, 2010, and Sept. 27, 2010, Stein he billed Blue Cross Blue Shield for 11 nasal endoscopies and 10 office outpatient visits for purported services rendered to J.F.

In truth, J.F. ceased seeing the doctor around September 3, 2010, and the doctor was in Germany from September 11, 2010 through September 27, 2010. The doctor received $725,156.45 from Blue Cross Blue Shield as a result of his submission of the false claims, and, under the plea agreement, agreed to pay restitution and forfeiture in the same amount.

A former nose surgeon from Northwest Indiana has been sentenced to seven years in prison for billing insurers and patients for procedures he didn't perform. This doctor, who ran a Merrillville nose and sinus clinic until he disappeared during a European vacation, pleaded guilty to 22 counts of health care fraud in a deal that called for a sentence of no more than of 10 years in prison. A prosecutor alleged that this doctor routinely performs diagnostic endoscopies on patients but bills these diagnostic procedures as more expensive and intrusive surgical debridement. Surgical debridements are a specialized procedure frequently performed following sinus surgery involving the trans nasal insertion of an endoscope and parallel insertion of various instruments to remove postsurgical crusting, bone or tissue deposits. It may also be used to remove crusts and debris in patients with longstanding chronic sinusitis who have undergone surgery in the past.

In addition to the allegations regarding surgical debridements, the case also involved the United States' allegations that the doctor systematically billed federal health benefit programs, in particular, Medicare and the Federal Employment Health Benefits Program, for claims arising from laryngeal video stroboscopies that were not performed or were not medically necessary.

"When physicians and their practices bill for services not provided or not medically necessary it undermines the public's trust in medical institutions and the financial integrity of federal health care programs," said Shimon R. Richmond, Special Agent in Charge, U.S. Department of Health and Human Services Office of Inspector General. "Our agents and lawyers will aggressively pursue those who exploit taxpayers, patients, and government health programs."

The ENT physician practicing in Plantation, Florida and his practice have agreed to pay $750,000 to resolve allegations that he violated the False Claims Act by billing for surgical endoscopies with debridement and laryngeal stroboscopies that were not provided or not medically necessary.

The court alleged that the doctor routinely performed diagnostic endoscopies on patients but billed these diagnostic procedures as more expensive and intrusive surgical debridement. Surgical debridements are a specialized procedure frequently performed following sinus surgery involving the transnasal insertion of an endoscope and parallel insertion of various instruments to remove postsurgical crusting, bone or tissue deposits. It may also be used to remove crusts and debris in patients with longstanding chronic sinusitis who have undergone surgery in the past.

Delaware's Division of Public Health (DPH) has ordered the closure of Delaware Otolaryngology Consultants, LLC, located at 17316 Coastal Highway, Lewes, Delaware 19958. Following complaints, the ear, nose, and throat medical practice was inspected by DPH and closed after the agency was unable to confirm that proper sterilization processes were followed. DPH encourages customers and employees who may have received services at this facility to contact their health care provider to discuss evaluation for diseases such as hepatitis and human immunodeficiency virus (HIV) that may have been transmitted through potentially unsterile equipment.

The doctor refused requests by BCBSNC to audit needed medical and billing records. As a result, the insurer filed a lawsuit asking the court to direct the doctor to cooperate with its request to audit records. The doctor's attorney responded to BCBSNC by filing a countersuit alleging that the insurer has withheld payments for medical claims submitted by this doctor including the same claims for which BCBSNC is seeking records. Following the doctor's countersuit, BCBSNC is seeking to amend its lawsuit, to allege claims for breach of contract, false and excessive billing, fraudulent misrepresentation and concealment, negligent misrepresentation, civil conspiracy, unfair and deceptive trade practices and state and federal Racketeer Influenced and Corrupt Organization Acts (RICO). The lawsuit seeks to recover compensatory and punitive damages as well.

Health care consumers need to identify these health care fraudsters and report them to attempt to salvage the health care system. People need to remember that he/she could receive a monetary reward for being a whistle blower.

Whistle blowers are people who expose unethical or illegal wrongdoing within companies by reporting it internally to superiors or externally to the media, government authorities, or specialized attorneys. They can be either current or past employees (insiders), or outside individuals who are familiar with the unlawful conduct, and are not required to be U.S. citizens. If you properly report Medicare fraud, you may be entitled to a significant whistleblower reward.

45. Pain Management Fraud

Pain management clinics specialize in treating chronic pain patients. Treatments involve therapy, injections, implantable devices and oral pain medications. Legitimate pain clinics have a trained certified clinician. Multiple fraudulent pain man management clinics exist and in some cases have become problematic. Pain patients need to investigate a clinic before they go to one because of fraudulent practices and practitioners in some clinics. Over a trillion dollars has been spent on healthcare and more than 4 billion health insurance claims were processed in the United States in 2011. Some of these health insurance claims were noted to be fraudulent. These fraudulent claims, however, result in higher premiums and out-of-pocket expenses for consumers. Healthcare fraud is committed by a small minority of healthcare providers.

Healthcare fraud consists of billing for services, which were never rendered or billing for expensive procedures that were never provided. Furthermore, performing medically unnecessary services to generate to insurance payments is another form of fraud as well. Falsification of a patient's diagnosis to justify surgeries, procedures or tests that aren't medically necessary also is fraudulent. Accepting kickbacks for patient referrals constitutes fraud and waving patient copayments also constitutes fraud under Medicare.

Healthcare fraud also involves making a false diagnosis of a medical condition that a patient does not have or describing more severe conditions then the patient actually has as well. Identity theft is also fraudulent. Doing unnecessary procedures also constitutes medical fraud. There are fraud and abuse allegations in interventional pain management practices as well. Furthermore, state investigators and state prosecutors have been targeting medical establishments that they believe may be operating as pill mills. It should be in noted that some pain physicians bill for patients that they have never seen even though prescriptions were written for narcotic medications.

Patients should be aware that some urine drug testing companies provide kickbacks to physicians who send urine drug screens to them. This is a serious offense and does some draw attention from the federal government with respect to fraud.

Most pain clinic's staff and are reputable and caring. However, many are not. For example, in 2009, insurance Corporate and Financial Investigations departments and law enforcement began receiving complaints about a doctor who claimed to specialize in pain management. One health insurance member in Michigan reported that his stolen insurance card had been used in the clinic by an individual trying to get narcotics. Another member said his wife had been contacted by a recruiter and told that she could get prescriptions for narcotics from this doctor. Other tenants at the medical office building where the practice was located complained to police about the crowds that were gathering in the parking lot and hallways of the building while individuals waited for hours to be seen by this doctor.

Joint investigation by the FBI, DEA, U.S. Department of Health and Human Services-Office of Inspector General and Blue Cross Blue Shield of Michigan revealed that patients were getting prescriptions for narcotics for no medical purpose. Patients were recruited to come to the office and agreed to diagnostic tests. In return, they would receive cash or prescriptions for hydrocodone, OxyContin, or Opana ER. Other patients agreed to get prescriptions for narcotics and then immediately turn them over to the recruiter. The recruiters were filling the prescriptions for resale on the streets.

In a typical visit, a patient would agree to medical tests such as blood tests, breathing tests, EKGs, EEGs, ultrasounds, X-rays, and psychological testing, no matter what their supposed medical problems were. All these tests were being billed to Blue Cross Blue Shield of Michigan and Medicare. The investigation revealed that for some of the tests that the clinic billed, the equipment was broken or the clinic did not even own the necessary equipment.

The doctor was initially charged in federal court with health care fraud. In a plea agreement, the doctor pled guilty to the charge of paying kickbacks. He was sentenced to 1 ½ years in jail, and his medical license was suspended. At the time of his arrest, the government seized $883,452 in assets from the doctor which he has since forfeited.

Patients who take Schedule II drugs are subject to random urine drug screens to valuate drug compliance and to ascertain that an individual is not taking a non-prescribed scheduled medication. If a patient takes a drug as prescribed, that drug will be present in the urine as his/her or her kidneys excrete the drug from the body. In Baltimore,

Maryland a federal grand jury indicted five defendants on charges arising from a scheme whereby physicians and administrative personnel associated with a Maryland pain management practice agreed to refer urine specimens to a testing lab for evaluation in return for $1.37 million in kickbacks:

Federal investigators said Thursday that a pharmaceutical sales manager helped organize a kickback scheme that paid tens of thousands of dollars in illicit fees to medical professionals in Connecticut and elsewhere who prescribed a powerful painkiller his employer manufactured. The payoff scheme probably cost the Medicare program millions of dollars by inducing physicians and other medical professionals to prescribe the painkiller to patients who were not eligible for the treatment under federal heath guidelines, authorities said.

FBI agents arrested a district sales manager for Arizona-based Insys Therapeutics, for paying kickbacks in relation to a federal health care program. His charges carry a sentence of up to five years. Pearlman, 49, of Edgewood, N.J., is accused of collecting a $95,000 quarterly bonus in 2013 based on his success selling Subsys, a powerful, fentanyl-based oral spray approved by the FDA to manage breakthrough pain experienced by cancer patients. Insys and Subsys were not mentioned by name in legal filings associated with the arrest, but multiple officials confirmed the identities.

This individual was accused in an FBI affidavit of arranging for $83,000 in kickbacks to just one Connecticut nurse who was authorized to write prescriptions by her ex-employer, the Comprehensive Pain and Headache Treatment Center of Derby. This individual an advanced practice nurse, is cooperating with federal investigators and was among the highest Subsys prescribers in the country.

Another individual has been charged with taking cancer drug kick-backs. Federal authorities said several of this physician's patients, who are Medicare Part D beneficiaries and who were prescribed the drug, did not have cancer, but were taking Subsys for chronic pain. Medicare and most private insurers will not pay for the drug unless the patient has an active cancer diagnosis, and an explanation that the drug is needed to manage the patient's cancer pain.

Federal prosecutors said that a company executive arranged hundreds of "sham" speakers programs to pay off doctors, and others qualified nurses for prescribing Subsys. The programs were ostensibly education gatherings to inform health professionals about pain management. In reality, federal officials said the programs were social gatherings at which Pearlman picked up the bill for food and drink and paid prescribers to attend.

The FBI said one drug company manager's sales territory was Connecticut, Rhode Island, New Jersey and New York and he arranged hundreds of speakers programs across the country. People involved in the investigation said it is continuing and that additional arrests are expected.

FBI agents arrested, a district sales manager for an Arizona-based Insys Therapeutics, for paying kickbacks in relation to a federal health care program. His charges carry a sentence of up to five years. One pharmaceutical company executive was accused of collecting a $95,000 quarterly bonus in 2013 based upon his success selling Subsys, a powerful, fentanyl-based oral spray approved by the FDA to manage breakthrough pain experienced by cancer patients. The sales manager was accused in an FBI affidavit of arranging for $83,000 in kickbacks to one Connecticut nurse who was authorized to write prescriptions by her ex-employer. A former Insys sales representative in Alabama also pleaded guilty to a conspiracy to violate the anti-kickback statute by paying two doctors to prescribe the drug. Illinois has filed claims against Insys related to pushing Subsys for unapproved uses.

The chief financial officer of a group of pain management clinics located in central Maryland was indicted. The group's clinics required its patients who have been prescribed pain relief medications to submit urine samples for testing in order to monitor the levels of pain medication or other narcotics in their bodies. The group's clinics generated hundreds of urine samples each month, which were sent to an outside lab for testing.

In March 2011, others at the group's clinics decided to shift the group's testing business to a laboratory testing company in New Jersey, after learning that the lab testing company was willing to pay a kickback for every urine sample that the group of clinics submitted for testing. The chief financial officer negotiated the arrangement, whereby the lab company promised to pay kickbacks equal to half of its profit, after accounting for expenses, for every urine sample that the group of clinics submitted for testing.

The group of clinics submitted urine samples for testing to the lab company from approximately March 2011 to August 2012. During this time, the lab company received total reimbursement payments of $4,033.846.70 from private insurers, Medicare and the Federal Employees Health Benefit Program for lab tests ordered by the group of clinics. Between the time the kickback payments commenced in July 2011 and the end of the scheme in July 2012, the lab company paid the group of clinics a total of $1,376,540.85 in kickbacks. Out of this amount, chief financial officer received approximately $459,245.

A New Jersey doctor admitted to hiding more than $3.6 million in income to avoid paying taxes and using the money to bribe other medical professionals for illegal pain referrals. He made up phony payroll expenses and hid money from his pain management business in private accounts, according to the state Division of Criminal Justice. This type of corruption in the health care industry, which causes patients to receive unnecessary services and raises costs for all healthcare consumers.

Pain management clinics specialize in treating chronic pain patients. Treatments involve therapy, injections, implantable devices and oral pain medications. Legitimate pain clinics have a trained board certified clinician in charge of the clinic as previously mentioned. Multiple fraudulent pain man management clinics have occurred and now exist and in some cases have become problematic. Pain patients need to investigate a clinic before going to a pain clinic because of fraudulent practices and practitioners.

Some pain clinics use a "hook em, stick em and boot em" pain treatment philosophy. A pain patient is initially hooked on pain pills, then ordered to have multiple pain injections and when the pain patient cannot afford more injections or the insurance will not pay any longer, the patient is dismissed (booted) from the practice.

Over one trillion dollars has been spent on healthcare and more than 4 billion health insurance claims were processed in the United States in 2011. Some of these health insurance claims were noted to be fraudulent. These fraudulent claims, however, carry an extremely high financial cost. Healthcare fraud results in higher premiums and out-of-pocket expenses for consumers. Healthcare fraud is committed by a small minority of healthcare providers.

Healthcare fraud consists of billing for services they were never rendered or billing for expensive procedures that were never provided. Furthermore performing medically unnecessary services to generate to insurance payments is another form of fraud as well. Falsification of a patient's diagnosis to justify surgeries, procedures, or tests that are not medically necessary also constitutes fraud.

Accepting kickbacks for patient referrals in most instances constitutes fraud. Furthermore, waving patient copayments to entice a patient into an office also constitutes fraud under Medicare. Healthcare fraud also involves making false diagnoses of a medical condition that a patient does not have or describing more severe conditions then the patient actually has as well. Identity theft is also fraudulent. A medical identity theft victim may unexpectedly be denied employment after a physical examination for potential employment because of a disease for which the person has never been diagnosed. Doing unnecessary procedures also constitutes medical fraud. There are fraud and abuse allegations in interventional pain management practices as well.

Furthermore, state investigators and prosecutors have been targeting medical establishments that they believe may be operating as pill mills. This occurs where patients with no pathology pay cash for narcotic prescriptions. It should be that some pain physicians bill for patients that they have never seen even though prescriptions were written for narcotic medications.

A patient should be aware that some urine drug testing companies provide kickbacks to physicians as well who send urine drug screens up to them for drug analysis. This is a serious offense and does some are draw attention from the federal government with respect to fraud. Pain doctors can charge more money if a pain procedure is done under X-ray or ultrasound needle guidance. There have been cases where patients have been placed under or in a "plain box" and were charged for x-ray utilization for pain block procedures when an x-ray machine or an ultrasound device was not actually used.

It is not illegal for a physician to prescribe narcotic drugs to patients who have no disease nor have no reason to have pain. This occurs when patients take prescriptions, get narcotics, and give the prescribing physician certain sums of money in return. The patient in many instances then sells the drugs on the street.

Health care consumers need to identify these health care fraudsters and report them to attempt to salvage the health care system. People need to remember that he/she could receive a monetary reward for being a whistle blower.

Whistle blowers are people who expose unethical or illegal wrongdoing within companies by reporting it internally to superiors or externally to the media, government authorities, or specialized attorneys. They can be either current or past employees (insiders), or outside individuals who are familiar with the unlawful conduct, and are not required to be U.S. citizens. If you properly report Medicare fraud, you may be entitled to a significant whistleblower reward.

46. Palliative Care Fraud

Palliative Care is a relatively new medical specialty. The goal of palliative care is to improve the quality of life for patients as well as their families. Palliative care is appropriate at any point in an illness. Palliative care can be provided at the same time as conventional treatment that is meant to cure you. Palliative care is dedicated to maximizing a person's comfort, independence, and quality of life when the prolongation of life is no longer a realistic goal. More than 50% of dying patients do not receive adequate symptomatic relief. Fear of hastening death is the primary reason for physicians' reluctance to prescribe high-dose pain medication.

Hospice became a Medicare benefit in 1983 for people with terminal conditions who had less than six months to live. A surge of public support eventually led to a government benefit that allowed patients to forgo heroic lifesaving measures in return for comfort measures and the opportunity to die at home. Medicare pays hospices about $154 a day for people with terminal medical problems who receive care at home, the most popular option. For providers, there are few quality standards to meet and no minimum requirements for how often to provide care.

Palliative care and hospice care are similar but different. Palliative care focuses on relief from physical suffering. The patient may be being treated for a disease or may be living with a chronic disease, and may or may not be terminally ill. It uses life prolonging medications. Hospice care makes the patient comfortable and prepares the patient and the patient's family for the patient's end of life when it is determined treatment for the illness will no longer be pursued. It does not use life-prolonging medications.

Hospice care is not designed to extend life, so the treatment offered is not intended to cure, but rather to provide comfort. Still, fewer patients have been dying within Medicare's six-month guideline. The principal incentive the hospice has is to keep its census high. For a hospice, death means money. From 1992 to 1998, the number of Medicare beneficiaries who used hospice care more than doubled, from 143,000 in 1992 to 360,000 in 1998. One of the areas under constant federal scrutiny is the length of time that patients stay in a hospice before they die. Hospices must be able to prove to regulators that the end was near for each patient.

No one knows how big the problem of hospice fraud is and all types of improper Medicare payments are estimated at $65 billion for 2010, but federal investigators prosecuted more than 60 cases in the last year alone, involving hundreds of millions of dollars nationwide. The system that was built to help dying patients live out their remaining days with dignity and comfort has few quality metrics to meet, no minimum requirements for how often care is provided, and low barriers to getting into the business. Critics say that can make end-of-life care seem ripe for abuse.

Palliative care is the active total care of patients whose disease is not amenable to curative treatment. Control of a patient's pain and other symptoms, and of psychological, social, and spiritual problems is mandatory. The goal is the achievement of the best possible quality of life for patients and their families. Palliative care aims to relieve symptoms such as pain, shortness of breath, fatigue, constipation, nausea, loss of appetite and difficulty sleeping. It helps patients gain the strength to carry on with daily life. It improves their ability to tolerate medical treatments. And it helps them better understand their choices for care. The goal of palliative care is to offer patients the best possible quality of life during their illness.

Palliative care is not the same as hospice care. Palliative care may be provided at any time during a person's illness, even from the time of diagnosis. And, it may be given at the same time as curative treatment. Hospice care always includes palliative care. However, it is focused on terminally ill patients-people who no longer seek treatments to cure them and who are expected to live for about six months or less. Palliative care affirms life and regards dying as a normal natural process. It neither hastens nor postpones death.

Palliative care provides relief from pain and psychological symptoms. Its goal is to integrate the psychological and spiritual aspects of a patient's care. It offers a support system to help patients live as actively as possible until their death. It offers a support system to help families cope during the patient's illness.

Palliative care is not provided by one physician but by a team of experts, including palliative care doctors, nurses and social workers. Chaplains, neuropaths, massage therapists, pharmacists, nutritionists and others are also a part of the team. Palliative care can be provided when you are at home, in an assisted-living facility, nursing facility or hospital. Palliative care in contrast to hospice care is not just for patients who are very close to death.

Palliative care is therefore, more than health care just for dying persons. Palliative care is a health care philosophy aimed at improving the essence of life when a cure is no longer possible. Palliative care is a health care discipline with its own research knowledge base, and a specific set of skills aimed at pain and other forms of suffering, which becomes the major focus of treatment.

A former hospice chief operating officer has been under indictment in federal court in Pittsburgh on charges of inflating enrollment at her company's facility by recruiting patients who often weren't really dying. In the Horizons case, prosecutors say the CEO. Stewart was pressuring her employees to recruit anyone they could find including people at bus stops in an inner-city. The goal was to keep the census high in order to bill Medicare and Medicaid for millions.

Federal prosecutors are seeking $202 million from a Wisconsin based care company where they allege nurses and other staff were instructed to increase hospice census "at all costs" and the mere suspicion of lung cancer was enough to enroll a patient for end of life care.

The American Board of Anesthesiology has subspecialty certification in palliative care. Palliative care is totally defined by prognosis but by what it inspires, offers, and achieves. A patient does not have to be dying to have palliative care. Palliative care is in addition to providing medical care, is also a provider of paramedical support services. Palliative care ensures informed choices be offered to patients.

The management of pain is an important aspect of palliative care. The patient must be regarded as a living person and therefore, the full human experiences; physical, emotional, and spiritual, must be addressed. A patient must not die with severe pain. The patient must be comfortable.

Most important a patient must be able to live out his or hers last moment as fully and consciously as possible. In fact, palliative care should make dying to be a patient's finest hour. A dying patient is unique and should be treated as someone special.

Palliative care is any form of medical care or treatment that concentrates on reducing the severity of disease symptoms rather than trying to seek a cure. The goal is to prevent and relieve suffering and to improve quality of life for people facing serious, complex illnesses. It should not be confused with hospice care which delivers palliative care to those at the end of life. In essence, palliative care provides care to those with life limiting illness at any stage of their disease.

Nutrition in palliative care and at the end of life should be one of the goals for improving quality of life. It is important to address issues of food and feeding during this time to assist in the management of troublesome sympatoms well as to enhance the remaining life. Cancer and its treatments exert a major impact upon physical and psychological reserves and at the end of life problems with appetite and the ability to eat and drink compound such impact.

Previous studies have shown that the dietary habits of cancer patients and survivors have significant implications for their recovery and quality of life. Nutrition and eating behaviors have a significant effect on cancer patients' physical and emotional adjustment. The aims of nutritional care minimize food-related discomfort and maximize food enjoyment. Ethical questions will be raised concerning the provision of food and fluids to a person nearing the end of his or her life. Nurses need to acknowledge that food has greater significance than the provision of nutrients.

The Office of Inspector General (OIG) has issued a special fraud alert, alerting the public to the high potential for fraud between hospices and nursing-home operators. Medicare provides palliative care in the form of hospice benefits to individuals who are terminally ill. That means the emphasis is on pain control, symptom management, and individualized counseling for not only the patient but her family too. The hospice must meet level and type of service requirements as well and have a written plan to fulfill them. Typical service requirements include physician and nursing services, speech, physical and occupational therapy, counseling and respite care as examples.

Although some of the core hospice services must be provided by the hospice directly to the beneficiary, others may be provided by other caregivers. However, all must be under the management of the hospice provider. The largest area for potential abuse in this cozy relationship between hospices and nursing homes stems from the nursing home's control over whom it will allow to provide hospice services in its facilities.

A hospice can derive substantial and recurring revenue if it has an ongoing exclusive contract to serve a large nursing home's patient base. This situation is ripe for the offer or request of financial kickbacks, incentives and other lucrative means to both parties. An OIG study showed that it's sometimes the case that nursing-home hospice patients receive fewer services than their home-bound counterparts. And since hospice providers are paid a flat rate, providing fewer services may positively affect their profitability and lessen their operating costs.

As in many health care fields, kickbacks are strictly prohibited by federal health care program, including Medicare and Medicaid. The ant kickback statute strictly prohibits the solicitation, receipt, offer or payment of "anything of value" to induce referrals of items or services payable by any federal health care program.

One particular area the OIG has observed as a potential source of abuse is when a hospice is paid a higher daily rate for a patient it refers to a nursing home. The law states that a hospice patient should be charged no more than if he had been enrolled as a non-hospice patient. Hospice patient referral to a nursing home as an inducement to the nursing home to its patients to the hospice is not legal.

In Metro Detroit, the arrested included six doctors, a social worker, a pharmacist and two physical therapists. According to officials, the schemes involved medical services that were unnecessary or never rendered, including hospice and home health care plus the billing, but not dispersal, of drugs. Authorities said the owners of home health care and hospice companies in Metro Detroit, two of whom are physical therapists, allegedly paid kickbacks to doctors and recruiters for referring patients to them, and then billed Medicare for unnecessary services.

In another case, the administrator and part owner of a hospice orchestrated an extensive scheme to fraudulently bill Medicare and Medicaid for millions of dollars by falsifying the level of hospice care provided for patients at nursing homes which he controlled. According to the charges, this administrator trained nurses to look for signs that allegedly would qualify a hospice patient for general inpatient care, resulting in payments per day more than four times higher than routine care rates. In many instances, patients were not terminally ill and wound up enrolled in hospice care far longer than the required life expectancy of six months or less.

In another case, the government contends that since at least 2007, a Texas-based hospice has fraudulently certified patients as terminally ill to illegally collect Medicare payments. The United States alleges that the hospice through its reckless business practices, admitted and retained individuals who were not eligible to receive Medicare hospice benefits, because it was financially lucrative and this hospice misspent millions of Medicare dollars intended for Medicare recipients."

In some instances, patients were admitted to hospice care, and then discharged just before the date at which the patient would reach the Medicare payment cap. That individual is then placed in the company's nursing-home facilities until that Medicare cap is reached, before being admitted once again to its hospice care. The government is increasing scrutiny on these fraudulent institutions and increasing the incidence of prosecution.

Health care consumers need to identify these health care fraudsters and report them to attempt to salvage the health care system. People need to remember that he/she could receive a monetary reward for being a whistle blower.

Whistle blowers are people who expose unethical or illegal wrongdoing within companies by reporting it internally to superiors or externally to the media, government authorities, or specialized attorneys. They can be either current or past employees (insiders), or outside individuals who are familiar with the unlawful conduct, and are not required to be U.S. citizens. If you properly report Medicare fraud, you may be entitled to a significant whistleblower reward.

47. Pathology Fraud

Pathology is the science of the causes and effects of diseases, especially the branch of medicine that deals with the laboratory examination of samples of body tissue for diagnostic or forensic purposes.

The marketing of pathology and laboratory services has become quite competitive in recent years, raising the compliance stakes with respect to marketing techniques in securing new clients and retaining existing clients. There is significant pressure on hospitals and health systems to pursue outreach opportunities, and because of the level of competition, some facilities have resorted to providing benefits to those providers who agree to direct business back to the facility.

However, any benefits provided to referral sources must be carefully considered in light of applicable federal and state fraud and abuse regulations, many of which carry criminal penalties in addition to substantial civil monetary fines. A typical hard-hitting analysis of an emerging clinical laboratory trend, it is noted that while these allegations are leveled at just a handful of lab companies, the amount of money these labs took out of the system exceeds a billion dollars, and some experts predict that payers will enact tough requirements to stop such abuses.

Pathologists and lab managers should not miss the point: this handful of bad actors within the lab industry accused of fraudulent business practices have taken more than $1 billion out of the healthcare system in just a couple of years! The total spent on clinical laboratory testing is about $75 billion per annum. The Office of the Inspector General (OIG) covers the provision of computers to referral sources of laboratory services. If the referral source is free to use the computer for a variety of purposes in addition to receiving test results, the provision of that computer may constitute an illegal inducement. The OIG also explains that the analysis would be equally applicable to fax or scanning machines, consulting services, or gifts given to referral sources, either for free or at a cost below fair market value.

The OIG explains that biopsy needles have a clear independent value to physicians and that the cost of the needles may already be included in the practice expense portion of the Medicare payment made to the physician. Under these circumstances, an obvious inference is that biopsy needles are being provided to the physicians by the pathology laboratories in exchange for referrals.

The OIG explains that a kickback violation can occur if the facility providing the lab services places a phlebotomist within the referral source's office or facility, and that individual performs clerical or medical functions not directly related to the collection or processing of laboratory specimens. This letter also describes as suspect the situation wherein a clinical laboratory provides a variety of chart review and infection-control services for nursing homes free of charge.

As fraud alert describes the following arrangements as suspect under the Medicare and Medicaid anti-kickback law: the provision, without charge, of a phlebotomist in a physician's office who performs additional tasks that are normally the responsibility of the physician's office staff (reiterating the OIG letter above); below-market laboratory pricing for renal dialysis centers; free pickup and disposal of biohazardous waste products unrelated to the collection of specimens for the outside laboratory; the provision of computers or fax machines without charge, unless such equipment is integral to and exclusively used for the performance of the outside laboratory's work; and provision of free laboratory testing for referring health care providers' employees and their families.

Much like the rest of the world, pathologists have been watching with fascination as the story of direct-to-consumer testing company Theranos unfolds. From the debut of its revolutionary "Edison machine" technology purportedly providing instant diagnoses from a single drop of blood to the discovery that not all was as it seemed, Theranos has been making headlines ever since it first caught the public's eye in 2013, a decade after its launch. But all that glitters is not diagnostic gold, and in 2015, the Wall Street Journal broke a story announcing that the company's flagship technology wasn't being used for most of its tests and that when it was used, the results might be inaccurate.

The Compassionate Care Hospice Group, Inc. has agreed to pay $2.4 million to resolve allegations that CCH Group and its subsidiary Compassionate Care Hospice of Atlanta, LLC, ("CCH Atlanta") submitted or caused the submission of false claims to Medicare and Medicaid by engaging in improper financial relationships with contracted physicians.

A North Carolina pathology practice has agreed to pay the U.S. $601,000 to settle a whistleblower's blower's False Claims Act lawsuit alleging it billed Medicare and Medicaid for medically unnecessary procedures. The U.S. Department of Justice said that the North Carolina practice was performing special tissue stain tests for diagnostic purposes before analyzing the routine hematoxylin, and eosin stain tests. The government considered the special tests costly and unnecessary because "a pathologist should review the specimen with the routine H&E stain before any special stain is used on the specimen," the Justice Department said.

Three individuals were charged with participating in a long-running scheme to bribe doctors to refer patient blood samples to a lab and to order unnecessary tests. This resulted action resulted in tens of millions of dollars in profit for the company. Between 2006 and 2013, these individuals and companies it funded paid millions of dollars to physicians in and around New Jersey to induce them to refer patient blood samples to the laboratory. From these referrals, this laboratory received tens of millions of dollars from private insurers and Medicare.

From 2007 to 2009, another laboratory director defrauded Medicare by submitting false and fraudulent claims for microbiology services never rendered when he owned and operated a pathology laboratory. The lab provided microbiology and other lab services. When the lab couldn't do certain types of microbiology testing, this company used another company that was not identified.

Generally, the laboratory submitted specimens to the unidentified company to test for infection-causing bacteria. Once an infection was found in a specimen, the unidentified company would run one or two more tests to identify the type of pathogen present and the type of antibiotic to which the pathogen was susceptible. This laboratory routinely billed Medicare for identification and susceptibility tests that were not actually done, even when initial testing showed no pathogen.

A whistle blower was a former laboratory contract salesperson for the practice who witnessed a program where the practice would provide Electronic Medical Record (EMR) software licenses to various physicians' practices in exchange for referrals. The government found that this laboratory provided EMR software licenses at little to no cost to nine physicians' practices close in time to when those practices entered contracts to refer specimens to their pathology lab. This conduct violated the Anti-Kickback Statute.

A North Carolina pathology practice has agreed to pay the U.S. $601,000 to settle a whistleblower's blower's False Claims Act lawsuit alleging it billed Medicare and Medicaid for medically unnecessary procedures used in the pathology laboratory practice.

The U.S. Department of Justice said that a pathology laboratory of Hickory, North Carolina, was performing special tissue stain tests for diagnostic purposes before analyzing the routine hematoxylin, and eosin (H&E) stain tests. The government considered the special tests costly and unnecessary because "a pathologist should review the specimen with the routine H&E stain before any special stain is used on the specimen.

The Department of Justice office is dedicated to ensuring that money is spent wisely on medically necessary services that benefit health care consumers as opposed to profiting on the bottom line of health care providers.

Health care consumers need to identify these health care fraudsters and report them to attempt to salvage the health care system. People need to remember that he/she could receive a monetary reward for being a whistle blower.

Whistle blowers are people who expose unethical or illegal wrongdoing within companies by reporting it internally to superiors or externally to the media, government authorities, or specialized attorneys. They can be either current or past employees (insiders), or outside individuals who are familiar with the unlawful conduct, and are not required to be U.S. citizens. If you properly report Medicare fraud, you may be entitled to a significant whistleblower reward.

48. Pediatric Fraud

Pediatrics is the treatment of children. Fraud may also be detected in the treatment of children as well as in other specialties. On February 25, 2009, the U.S. Department of Justice released a complaint against New York-based Forest Laboratories and their fraudulent practices in marketing the medications Celexa and Lexapro. Forest allegedly promoted the drugs for unapproved pediatric use and paid kickbacks to physicians who prescribed them. The illegal practices prompted the submission of thousands of false claims to federal healthcare programs.

The complaint, filed by numerous parties, claims that Forest actively marketed the drugs for pediatric use despite the FDA's denial of a pediatric indication. It was alleged that a "double-blind, placebo-controlled, pediatric trial" deemed Celexa of no greater value than the placebo for pediatric use, and; furthermore, patients using Celexa recorded more suicide attempts and suicidal thoughts than the group using the placebo. Despite the study results, Forest continued the promotion of the drugs and deceived physicians and the public by failing to disclose the negative findings.

The United States has alleged that health care programs paid thousands of false claims for Celexa and Lexapro prescriptions that were not covered for off-label pediatric use and were ineligible for payments due to illegal kickbacks. Forest allegedly attempted to induce physicians through expensive dinners, sumptuous entertainment, and various methods of illegal payment, including bribes masked as consulting fees or grants. All of these come in violation of the federal anti-kickback statute.

The former owner of a Nashville pediatric practice has pled guilty to health care fraud and was ordered to pay $1.6 million in restitution and damages. The sale of Centennial Pediatrics, another requirement of the plea agreement, was completed on Oct. 31. The doctor was charged with billing for infant hearing exams that he did not have equipment capable of performing. He acknowledged billing for tests that would only be found necessary through microscopic examinations when his clinics had no microscopes. Investigations are part of increased efforts during recent years to investigate possible fraud among health providers who are paid to treat poor children and the disabled.

A former administrative worker at a Florida-based pediatric practice has been indicted in federal court along with two others for alleged identity theft and fraud crimes involving stolen patient information. "It was a part of the conspiracy that the conspirators and others would, and did, steal and obtain stolen personally identifiable information from various sources. This stolen information included names, dates of birth, and Social Security numbers, among other things, of a medical practice's current and former patients, patients' parents and patients' guardians, indictment document notes.

Federal prosecutors say the conspirators, using the stole information electronically applied for credit cards and lines of credit to Discover, Capital One, and other financial services firms, and then used or attempted to use the unauthorized credit cards to purchase items from retailers and withdraw cash from ATMs. Additionally, prosecutors allege that the stolen patient information was used to file fraudulent federal income tax returns in an attempt to obtain tax refunds.

The Department of Health and Human Services' Office for Civil Rights appears to have closed an investigation into a pediatric incident, which listed a tally of major breaches as affecting 13,000. A recent case involving a former Tampa General Hospital worker who was sentenced on Aug. 3 to 37 months in federal prison on HIPAA violations and tax fraud charges (see HIPAA Criminal Prosecutions on Rise).

The factors prosecutors weigh in deciding whether to pursue HIPAA violations in fraud cases involving patient information can vary based on a number of considerations. Studies have shown a persistent threat from unauthorized disclosure of patient information by insiders, whether it be stalking, snooping or using patient financial information for financial crimes.

Organizations are advised to take action to perform a background investigation of workforce members who have access to patient information and financial information. Use software applications to monitor activity of those who have access to patient records, including contractors and outsiders given access to your organization's information systems. Employees have access to sensitive data and are a significant risk.

The State of Vermont and Mousetrap Pediatrics PC, have reached an agreement settling an investigation into whether Mousetrap submitted false claims or received overpayments from the Vermont Medicaid Program. Mousetrap operated as a pediatric physician group for over twenty-five years in the Franklin County area, until its dissolution in January 2016.

The settlement resolves an investigation into Mousetrap's Medicaid claims related to after-hours office visits. The investigation revealed that from January 28, 2013, through December 7, 2015, Mousetrap submitted claims to Medicaid using an improper billing code for services provided during regularly scheduled extended office hours. Mousetrap received $51,553.65 more from the Vermont Medicaid program than it would have been entitled had the claims been properly submitted. The improper use of the billing code was caused by a change in Mousetrap's business practices regarding extended offices hours, and not due to any intentional fraudulent behavior. MFRAU found that Mousetrap's use of the code prior to January 28, 2013 did not violate any Medicaid or coding rules.

Mousetrap will pay $66,553.65 to settle potential claims under the Vermont False Claims Act. Under the settlement agreement, Mousetrap will repay the Medicaid Program the $51,553.65 it improperly received and a $15,000.00 civil penalty. The settlement followed an investigation by the Medicaid Fraud and Residential Abuse Unit of the Office of the Attorney General and the Program Integrity Unit of the Department of Vermont Health Access.

A provider of home nursing services for severely disabled children has agreed to pay over $2.7 million to settle allegations that it failed to return overpayments it received from state Medicaid programs and federally-insured health programs, and overcharged for home nursing services. The settlement with Georgia-based company, Pediatric Services of America, Inc., (PSA), was joined by 19 other states and the federal government to resolve civil allegations that the company unlawfully withheld overpayments and overcharged for nursing services by improperly rounding-up claims to the nearest whole hour.

Fraud may also occur with respect to vaccines. According to the US Food and Drug Administration, safety assessments for vaccines have not often included toxicity studies because vaccines have not been viewed as inherently toxic. However, vaccines are legally defined as unavoidably unsafe.

Most people in the U.S. do not know that U.S. law prevents anyone damaged by vaccines from suing the manufacturer. In 1986, there were so many lawsuits resulting from vaccine injuries and deaths prior to this time, that it was no longer profitable for pharmaceutical companies to continue marketing vaccines without legal protection. So instead of Congress requiring that drug companies manufacture safer vaccines, they complied with the drug companies' requests and passed legislation protecting the drug companies. In 2011, this law was upheld by the U.S. Supreme Court.

A lawsuit was brought by two whistle blowers, who were virologists who worked for Merck and were accusing Merck of lying about the effectiveness of the mumps vaccine. There was also a class-action suit related, brought by Alabama-based Chatom Primary Care and two individual doctors from New York and New Jersey that allege Merck's monopoly on the drug caused them to pay more for the drug.

It is not just childhood vaccines that come with substantial risk. Influenza vaccines, vaccines for sexually transmitted diseases, and others contain similar risks for adverse events. Also troubling is that vaccination is recommended now for pregnant women, even though vaccine package inserts clearly state they have not been tested on pregnant women, so the effects on the fetus can't be known.

In the 1960s only a handful of childhood vaccines were given. The current CDC recommended vaccine schedule for children now has over 30 vaccines by the time a child turns 6 and an additional potential for up to 30 more by the time they reach 18 years of age.

Since genetic mutations change slowly over generations, we must look to environmental causes for these changes. While other environmental toxins certainly are at play in these statistics, disregarding the potential role to the amounts of toxin injected into children through vaccines is not only bad public policy, it is bad science. By disregarding the role of vaccines in our statistics for infant mortality and chronic diseases, we could be doing more harm than good in mandating, or even advising, then.

Vaccines are known to be problematic for a segment of the population with a specific mitochondrial genetic mutation which may affect up to 4,000 babies a year. Some of those with a particular form of this dysfunction are unable to detoxify the poisons such as aluminum or mercury that are in the vaccine. This inability to detoxify the metals causes damage to multiple organ systems with sometimes devastating results.

Mercury, another heavy metal and known neurotoxin, is in all inactivated flu vaccines where it is used as a preservative in the form of thimerosal. Though thimerosal is no longer used as a preservative in childhood vaccines, it remains present in them in in trace amounts since it is part of the manufacturing process. However, those trace amounts still exceeds the FDA recommended amounts that can be ingested. Vaccines are injected rather than ingested. The mainstream media seems united in their belief that vaccines do not cause harm, and that the rise of childhood diseases is due to unvaccinated children, rather than faulty vaccines.

Despite lack of support by the medical and scientific community, chiropractic treatment of children is growing in popularity, and more chiropractors are specializing in chiropractic pediatrics. Studies are beginning to show that chiropractic can help children with issues as varied as asthma, chronic ear infections, nursing difficulties, colic and bedwetting.

To date, legitimate properly-controlled studies have failed to support the claims of chiropractors who treat children for organic ailments. Although otitis media is normally self-limiting, it should be kept under observation by a pediatrician who can prescribe antibiotics, if needed. Because of the damage that manipulation might do to cartilaginous growth centers, there is no known justification for using spinal manipulation on an infant or a pre-adolescent child.

When back pain as a child does occur, it is potentially more serious than back pain in an adult and should always be brought to the attention of a board-certified pediatrician. A systematic review of 13 studies published up to June 2004 uncovered 14 significant manipulation-related injuries in children up to 18 years of age, 9 of which were serious (e.g., subarachnoidal hemorrhage, paraplegia) and 2 of which were fatal (one child died from a brain hemorrhage and another from dislocation of the atlas following neck manipulation). Ten of the injuries were attributed to manipulation done by chiropractors, 1 to manipulation by a physiotherapist, and 1 to manipulation by a medical doctor; two injuries were caused by unspecified providers of manipulation.

Pediatric chiropractic care is often inconsistent with recommended medical guidelines. Although spinal manipulation is often recommended as a treatment for back pain, this recommendation does not often apply to children.

A pediatrician knowingly up coded billings for infant auditory screening exams to Tennessee's Medicaid program and commercial insurance programs. Specifically, Centennial billed for the infant hearing exams that it performed at Baptist Hospital as comprehensive auditory exams, even though it only performed the less expensive auditory screens. The investigation revealed that Centennial did not even have equipment capable of performing the comprehensive tests for which it billed.

Furthermore, according to the plea agreement, the pediatrician admitted that through numerous Centennial clinics, he systemically billed for urinalysis testing as though its office had performed a microscopic examination of the sample despite the fact that no microscopy had been performed. Centennial up coded its billings in this manner even though its clinics did not own or possess the microscopes necessary to conduct such examinations.

Health care consumers need to identify these health care fraudsters and report them to attempt to salvage the health care system. People need to remember that he/she could receive a monetary reward for being a whistle blower.

Whistle blowers are people who expose unethical or illegal wrongdoing within companies by reporting it internally to superiors or externally to the media, government authorities, or specialized attorneys. They can be either current or past employees (insiders), or outside individuals who are familiar with the unlawful conduct, and are not required to be U.S. citizens. If you properly report Medicare fraud, you may be entitled to a significant whistleblower reward.

49. Physical Medicine Fraud

Physical Medicine and Rehabilitation (PM&R), also known as physiatry or rehabilitation medicine, or physical and rehabilitation medicine is a branch of medicine that aims to enhance and restore functional ability and quality of life to those with physical impairments or disabilities. A physician having completed training in this field is referred to as a physiatrist. Physiatrists specialize in restoring optimal function to people with injuries to the muscles, bones, ligaments, or a patient's nervous system.

Dallas County Hospital District d/b/a Parkland Health and Hospital System (Parkland) settled allegations it violated the civil False Claims Act and Texas Medicaid Fraud Prevention Act. The U.S. and Texas contend Parkland caused unallowable and "up coded"" physician consultations and other services to be submitted to Medicare and Texas Medicaid for certain physical medicine and rehabilitation (PMR) related items and services between 2007 and 2011. Parkland fully cooperated with the investigation, and by settling, did not admit any wrong-doing or liability.

When patients are admitted to a hospital, specialists, like PMR physicians, often consult with the attending physician on a variety of issues. At teaching hospitals, faculty physicians may bill for the supervision of residents, if present for the key or critical portions of the services. In both cases such consults, if medically appropriate, are reimbursed by Medicare and Texas Medicaid.

The United States and Texas based their investigation on allegations that Parkland submitted or caused the submission of false and fraudulent PMR claims, and false statements in support of such claims, to the Medicare and Texas Medicaid programs between 2007 and 2011 for: (1) consultations that were never requested by a patient's treating physicians and/or lacked medical necessity; (2) services related to the inappropriate supervision of residents and/or lacked medical necessity; (3) up-coded and inflated evaluation and management services; (4) inpatient rehabilitation stays that did not meet billing requirements; and (5) other unreimbursable costs.

According to another indictment and documents filed in court, an individual was a physician specializing in physical medicine and rehabilitation. She was a participating provider in Medicare and Medicaid. Most of her patients were Medicare and Medicaid beneficiaries. She was the sole owner and CEO of a physical medicine and rehabilitation practice in Minnesota that specialized in pain management and rehabilitation.

According to the indictment and documents filed in court, from at least February 2011 through December 2014, this doctor conspired with others to fraudulently bill Medicare and Medicaid for topical pain-relief creams that she prescribed. The defendant referred virtually every patient prescribed topical pain-relief cream to a single pharmacy which prepared and dispensed the topical pain-relief creams.

According to the indictment and documents also filed in court, a pharmacist at the pharmacy in question who was also charged separately by information, compounded pain creams using bulk-powder forms of the various ingredients called for by the prescriptions and dispensed in the pain creams to customers. This pharmacy then submitted claims for reimbursement to Medicare and Medicaid that falsely represented that the pain creams had been made using tablet, capsule or liquid forms of the various ingredients in the pain creams. By including these false representations, the pharmacy generated inflated reimbursements on the pain creams. In exchange for the doctor referring all the prescriptions for these pain creams to the one pharmacy, the pharmacy paid the doctor more than $40,000 in kickbacks. According to the indictment the doctor also knowingly wrote prescriptions, on at least one occasion, for morphine and oxycodone in the absence of a legitimate medical purpose and outside the course of usual professional practice.

In another case a physical medicine and rehabilitative specialist currently practicing in Alabama and a local neurosurgeon physician group, agreed collectively to pay $1.4 million to resolve allegations, they violated the False Claims Act by billing federal health care programs for medically unreasonable and unnecessary ultrasound guidance used with routine lab blood draws, and with Botox and trigger point injections. As a result of this billing scheme, the defendants sometimes billed 15 to 30 identical ultrasound guidance claims for a single patient office visit.

A licensed Mississippi physician was arrested in December for fraudulently billing the federal government $16 million for in-home physical therapy services, according to the HHS Office of Inspector

General. The indictment, filed Dec. 3, 2008, alleges that the doctor received $7 million in unjustified payments.

A physician and owner and operator of a physical medicine practice were charged with conspiracy, healthcare fraud, making false statements, theft of public money, and wire fraud, the OIG reported. According to an indictment, the so-called physical therapy services were provided in patients' homes by unqualified, inadequately trained, unlicensed technicians with no supervision and then billed as though the doctor had provided or supervised the services.

Seven people associated with a medical clinic have been indicted for alleged Medicaid and Medicare fraud, and federal authorities seized millions of dollars in cash and property in Mississippi and Texas, court records said.

A physical medicine and rehabilitation billed Medicare and Medicaid for more than $39 million in services in Mississippi during the alleged conspiracy, from 2000 to 2005, according to the indictment. The government agencies paid out $18 million. It's not clear how much of that was obtained by allegedly fraudulent billing. The government has seized more than $3.6 million from various accounts and prosecutors are seeking the forfeiture of three properties, one each in the Texas towns of Cedar Hill and Spring, and one in Ellisville, Miss.

The alleged scheme took place in Mississippi through a clinic that "purported to provide in-home physical therapy services," according to the 19-page indictment. At least four of those indicted are doctors who once worked as medical directors for Statewide Physical Medicine Group, according to the 13-count indictment, dated Oct. 20. Three others owned or operated the company at one time. The defendants are accused of conspiring to make fraudulent claims, billing for services that were not provided by a doctor or under the direct supervision of a doctor, inflating the time they spent with patients, and lying to patients about having to make co-payments for services.

Health care consumers need to identify these health care fraudsters and report them to attempt to salvage the health care system. People need to remember that he/she could receive a monetary reward for being a whistle blower.

Whistle blowers are people who expose unethical or illegal wrongdoing within companies by reporting it internally to superiors or externally to the media, government authorities, or specialized attorneys. They can be either current or past employees (insiders), or

outside individuals who are familiar with the unlawful conduct, and are not required to be U.S. citizens. If you properly report Medicare fraud, you may be entitled to a significant whistleblower reward.

50. Psychiatry Fraud

The United States loses approximately $100 billion to health care fraud each year. Up to $20 billion of this is due to fraudulent practices within the mental health industry. One of the largest health care fraud suits in US history was in mental health, yet it is the smallest sector within health care. A study of US Medicaid and Medicare insurance fraud, especially in New York, over a twenty-year period, showed psychiatry to have the worst track record of all medical disciplines.

Investigators routinely find psychiatrists responsible for a disproportionate share of the fraud and corruption within the health care industry. Florida Medicare investigators found that 40 percent of all mental health outpatient service billings in 1994 were fraudulent. As far back as 1985, a U.S. Justice Department probe found that while psychiatrists represented only 8 percent of the physicians in the country, they accounted for 18 percent of the crooked doctors suspended from Medicaid programs over a 15-year period the worst performance of any group in the medical field.

Crimes included charging for therapy when they had only doled out drugs; billing for patients who did not exist; falsely billing for up to 24 hours of therapy per day; and having sex with patients and billing the government for their lust. Florida Medicare investigators found that 40 percent of all mental health outpatient service billings in 1994 were fraudulent.

A February 1985 article in the American Journal of Psychiatry said, "Psychiatrists may also cheat more than other doctors because they find the benefit system, particularly unresponsive to what they consider to be their fiscal due." The atrocities of Johnson and Johnson, in collaboration with the psychiatry fraud have occurred and it is important to realize that they are by no means the only ones. Pharmaceutical companies, who manufacture highly toxic drugs to treat every one of these "disorders," are leading the charge to invent more and more mental-health categories, so they can sell more drugs and make more money.

The United States loses approximately $100 billion to healthcare fraud each year. Up to $40 billion of this is due to fraudulent practices within the mental health industry. At least 10 percent of psychiatrists admit to sexually abusing their patients. Some studies estimate that the figure is as high as 25 percent, and a California study claims 48 percent. All studies estimate that a vast majority of these rapes go unreported.

The Citizens Commission on Human Rights International (CCHR) is a Scientology front group that campaigns against psychiatry and psychiatrists. CCHR's database of mental health criminal convictions (which is by no means complete) numbers over 1,300 convictions worldwide over the last 30 years for everything from theft and drunk driving to rape, manslaughter and murder.

In 2012 global health care giant GlaxoSmithKline agreed to plead guilty and to pay $3 billion to resolve it's criminal and civil liability arising from the company's unlawful promotion of mostly psychiatric drugs. In the same Abbot Laboratories, had to pay out $1.5 billion, including 700 million in criminal fines and forfeitures, again for the unapproved promotion of psychiatric 'medication'. In all cases, the common linking factor is the psychiatric drug trade.

The mental health monopoly has practically zero accountability and zero liability for its failures. This has allowed psychiatrists and psychologists to commit far more than just financial fraud. The roster of crimes committed by these "professionals" ranges from fraud, drug offenses, rape and sexual abuse to child molestation, assault, manslaughter and murder. Pharmaceutical companies, who manufacture highly toxic drugs to treat every one of these "disorders," are leading the charge to invent more and more mental-health categories, so they can sell more drugs and make more money.

The Fourth Edition of the Diagnostic and Statistical Manual of Mental Disorders, or DSM IV is the standard classification of mental disorders used by mental health professionals in the United States. It used for patient diagnosis and treatment, and is important for collecting and communicating accurate public health statistics. The DSM IV allowed for more toxic drugs to be prescribed, because the definitions of bipolar and ADHD were expanded to include more people. Adverse effects of Valproate (given for a bipolar diagnosis) include: acute, life-threatening, and even fatal liver toxicity; life-threatening inflammation of the pancreas; and brain damage.

Some adverse effects of Lithium (also given for a bipolar diagnosis) include: intracranial pressure increases leading to blindness;

peripheral circulatory collapse; stupor and coma. Adverse effects of Risperdal (given for "Bipolar" and "irritability stemming from autism") include: serious impairment of cognitive function; fainting; restless muscles in neck or face, tremors (may be indicative of motor brain damage).

The Department of Justice alleged Park Avenue Medical Associates billed for psychiatry services for patients whose dementia or cognitive disorders actually made them unable to benefit from psychotherapy. Authorities also charged the company with billing for services where there was no documentation. PAMA billed for nearly 91,000 exams that "were duplicative, failed to comply with Medicare rules and reflected a lack of coordination of care both among PAMA's own psychiatrist, psychologists and nurses, and between PAMA"s employees and staff at the facilities at which PAMA performed services," according to the complaint. Prosecutors said the organization gave incentives to employees to "perform unnecessary and duplicative services by compensating them based on how many services they provided and the level at which Medicare reimbursed for those services." It continued that PAMA's compliance program was "inadequate" to detect and counter the illegal billings.

The evidence presented at trial showed that individuals participated in a scheme by which a psychological unit paid bribes and kickbacks to group home owners and nursing-home employees in exchange for sending Medicare patients to the psychological unit. The psychiatrist in charge indiscriminately admitted and readmitted these patients into these intensive psychiatric programs often for years on end many of whom suffered from severe Alzheimer's or dementia and were unable to participate in the treatment purportedly provided at the PHPs, and who therefore did not qualify for the services, the evidence showed.

In addition, evidence presented at trial showed that the psychiatrist rarely saw patients, and that he visited the psychiatric units briefly every week or so to sign documents and briefly see patients. Additionally, he falsified medical records and signed false documents purporting to show that patients admitted to the psychiatric unit qualified and required the intensive psychiatric services, the evidence showed.

Evidence also showed that the unit did not actually provide the intensive, psychiatric treatment that a psychiatrical unit is supposed to provide and falsified documentation to make it appear to Medicare that intensive treatment was being provided to qualifying patients. Evidence at trial demonstrated that the psychiatrist personally billed Medicare for over $4.5 million for psychiatric treatment he purportedly provided to the psychiatric patients.

When you look below the surface at the specialty of psychiatry what you uncover is so preposterous it is difficult to believe that it is really true. Prominent psychiatrists from all over the world gather annually for a meeting at which new diseases are invented. There are no objective findings that establish the diagnosis of these diseases.

These new diseases are included in the Diagnostic and Statistical Manual of Mental Diseases. Potential new diseases are discussed during these meetings, and new diseases are voted in or out by a show of hands. Among the new diseases are social anxiety disorder (everyone who is uncomfortable in a social setting has this disease) and mathematics disease (anyone who has struggled over a math problem has this disease).

Gender identity disorder, passive-aggressive disorder, disorder of written expression and sexual disorder are other examples of invented diseases that will follow the individuals tagged with these diagnoses the remainder of their lives. Naturally, all these phony diseases have a psychoactive drug which supposedly ameliorates this disease.

When a child is diagnosed with depression, the child is often placed on a potent SSRI drug. The manufacturer of one of the leading SSRI drugs knew for many years that the drug caused loss of the ability to control violent behavior thus increasing violence toward self (suicide) and others (mass murders). This information was covered up because it would have hurt sales of the drug. Nearly every teen involved in the Columbine, and Red Lake mass murders was taking an SSRI drug.

In June 2003, a psychiatrist filed a lawsuit against Pennsylvania officials and several drug companies. This doctor was hired by the Pennsylvania Bureau of Program Integrity in the Department of Public Welfare to oversee mental health and substance abuse programs. In this position, he uncovered serious abuses, including the deaths of four children and one adult while in state custody due to substandard care and the misuse of psychiatric drugs and also the sexual abuse of children by staff personnel. His suit also says drug companies have "distorted statistics, violated regulations and misrepresented the effects of the use of their psychotropic drugs simply to make money."

In May 2002 Northwestern Human Services, a Pennsylvania mental health services company, agreed to pay $7.8 million to the government to resolve civil claims that the company submitted false and fraudulent bills to Medicare and Medicaid, seeking reimbursement for mental health services. The civil charges included billing for patients who were so impaired that they were unable to participate in the program; billing for services that were simply recreational in nature; submitting false records of psychiatric time spent with each patient and causing staff and others to pose as clinical staff members during annual inspections by the Department of Public Welfare to demonstrate compliance with the staffing requirements.

Health care consumers need to identify these health care fraudsters and report them to attempt to salvage the health care system. People need to remember that he/she could receive a monetary reward for being a whistle blower.

Whistle blowers are people who expose unethical or illegal wrongdoing within companies by reporting it internally to superiors or externally to the media, government authorities, or specialized attorneys. They can be either current or past employees (insiders), or outside individuals who are familiar with the unlawful conduct, and are not required to be U.S. citizens. If you properly report Medicare fraud, you may be entitled to a significant whistleblower reward.

51. Pulmonology Fraud

Pulmonology is known as chest medicine and respiratory medicine in some countries and areas. Pulmonology is considered a branch of internal medicine, and is related to intensive care medicine. Pulmonology often involves managing patients who need life support and mechanical ventilation. Pulmonologists are specially trained in diseases and conditions within the chest, particularly pneumonia, asthma, tuberculosis, emphysema, and complicated chest infections.

From October 2008 to December 2009, a pulmonary doctor devised a scheme to defraud the Medicare program by hiring unlicensed individuals to perform services that were billed to Medicare as respiratory therapy services and by instructing her staff to falsify records setting forth the amount of time during which services were provided. She also instructed employees to designate certain services for billing under physical therapy codes, which resulted in payments approximately double those of respiratory codes, and instructed employees to designate certain services to be double or triple billed using both physical therapy and respiratory therapy codes, even though Pulmonary Solutions never employed any physical therapists. In total, this doctor caused fraudulent claims in excess of $1,000,000 to be paid by Medicare and Medicaid for fraudulently billed respiratory therapy services.

By copying old information into patient records, a pulmonologist at a Veterans hospital may have committed insurance fraud, according to an internal VA report on the case. The Department of Veterans Affairs own medical inspector said the pulmonologist's actions might amount to falsification of a government document. If third-party payers were billed for any of the pulmonologist's medical evaluations based on copied and pasted entries into the medical record, this could constitute fraud, according to the initial 2013 report from the VA's Office of the Medical Inspector.

The VA bills private health insurance providers for medical care, supplies and prescriptions to treat veterans' conditions unrelated to their military service. After the medical inspector's initial report, further investigation found the pulmonologist at the Montgomery campus of Central Alabama Veterans Health Care System copied old information from patient records more than 1,200 times from 2011 to 2013, according to the U.S. Office of Special Counsel. The counsel's office ordered the review based on information provided by a whistle-blower.

The initial report, a copy of which was released by Congress with names blacked out, said the pulmonologist admitted to copying and pasting data gathered by other doctors such as patient history, vital signs, examinations, assessments and plans of care, into his own assessments. He acknowledged, in his words, that his 'technical incompetence' and 'stupidity' resulted in the inclusion of other's information in his signed notes. The case of the Montgomery pulmonologist has figured prominently in the national scandal over how long veterans have to wait to see a VA doctor, attempts to cover up the long wait times and how the delays affect patient health.

The government recently entered into a settlement agreement with home oxygen and respiratory medications equipment and services company regarding a False Claims Act lawsuit that was filed against the company in 2010. The lawsuit alleges that the company engaged in government programs fraud by incentivizing physicians to conduct tests and prescribe sleep therapy and oxygen products to patients who utilize government health insurance programs such as Medicare, Medical (California's Medicaid program), and TRICARE, that were medically unnecessary. The company was founded in Bakersfield, California in 1978 and currently operates in over 16 states across the country. PPS supplies home oxygen therapy products to patients, as well as sleep therapy equipment and nebulized medications to treat respiratory conditions such as Chronic Obstructive Pulmonary Disease. Under this scheme, the company was able to submit false claims to the government for payment for the products and services that were gratuitously administered. The company has agreed to settle the allegations for $11.4 million.

A Pennsylvania pulmonologist and the sole owner of Central Pennsylvania Pulmonary Associates (CPPA) and Sleep Disorder Centers of Central Pennsylvania in June 2012 and again in July, Clark was indicted by a federal grand jury in Harrisburg in separate indictments. In June 2012, the doctor was indicted on charges that from July 2010 through December 2011, as the owner of CPPA, and the trustee of the CPPA employee 401(k) Plan, he withheld employee 401(k) contributions and failed to deposit the withheld funds into their 401(k) Plan. The doctor instead maintained the employee 401(k) contributions in bank accounts he controlled. The employees lost approximately $25,000 of their retirement funds.

In July 2012, the doctor was indicted on charges that from December 2007 through September 26, 2008. The doctor, who provided critical care services to patients of Holy Spirit Hospital, intentionally inflated the amount of time the healthcare providers he employed spent with each patient, thereby fraudulently inflating the health insurance claims that the doctor submitted to Medicare, Highmark, Inc., and Capital Blue Cross. The dollar amount of the fraudulent claims exceeded $500,000. In the indictment's six money laundering counts were identified, and the doctor was charged with transferring approximately $103,000 obtained through the healthcare fraud to CPPA payroll and money-market accounts.

The Medicare Modernization Act of 2003 established the Medicare Recovery Audit Contractor (RAC) program to identify fraud and waste in the Medicare system. The California Medical Association (CMA) has recently learned that RAC contractor Health Data Institute (HDI) is currently assessing overpayments for evaluation and management services billed without a modifier 25 on the same day as a diagnostic pulmonary study. Affected claims have dates of service of 2009 or 2010.

In order for a physician to receive payment for a visit on the same day as a service in the pulmonary diagnostic range, the physician must append a modifier 25 with the visit code, indicating that the patient's condition required a significant, separately identifiable visit above and beyond the diagnostic service provided.

Increasing numbers of troubled sleepers are seeking diagnosis and treatment of chronic sleep disorders that affect more than fifty million Americans. The significant growth in sleep medicine over recent years brings increasing opportunities for the unscrupulous to engage in fraudulent services and billing. The most common method of diagnosing sleep disorders is a polysomnography test, which involves the monitoring and assessing of physiological reactions during sleep. Results of this test might show, for example, the presence of obstructive sleep apnea (OSA). A diagnosis of OSA often leads to a prescription for a continuous positive airway pressure (CPAP) device, which keeps the patient's airway open and unobstructed during sleep.

Medicare spending on polysomnography services is extremely high: $407 million in 2005, increasing to $565 million in 2011. With the uptick in sleep disorder services and government spending comes the discovery of various schemes that defraud federal and state health care programs that reimburse for such services.

Medicare, Medicaid, and other government programs reimburse claims for sleep tests and devices that are "reasonable and necessary" or "medically necessary" and impose a number of related requirements. For example, Medicare reimbursement requires that sleep tests be conducted by physicians or properly licensed or certified sleep technologists.

Sleep tests also must be performed under the appropriate level of doctor supervision, including overall direction and control. Moreover, independent diagnostic testing facilities (e.g., non-hospital based sleep test centers), must be properly enrolled and approved by Medicare on a location-by-location basis. A provider who knowingly fails to meet these requirements yet bills a government program might be violating the False Claims Act.

Another area of potential abuse is the prescribing and dispensing of durable medical equipment (DME) such as CPAP devices. Knowingly prescribing and seeking reimbursement for devices without demonstrating the proper need defrauds government health care programs. As with independent diagnostic sleep study facilities, each location of a DME supplier must be in an appropriate site that is separately enrolled and approved by Medicare. Moreover, DME, with its individual sizing and pressure settings, must be dispensed by properly qualified personnel.

Federal laws and regulations also prohibit certain self-interested dealing or business-overlap between sleep-test providers and device suppliers. Branden Partners, L.P., doing business as Pacific Pulmonary Services, agreed to pay $11.4 million to resolve allegations that it and its general partner, Teijin Pharma USA LLC, and violated the False Claims Act. Pacific Pulmonary Services provides oxygen tanks and related supplies, and sleep therapy equipment, to patients' homes.

The allegations were that, starting in 2004; Pacific Pulmonary Services began submitting claims for reimbursement to Medicare and other federal healthcare programs for home oxygen and oxygen equipment without obtaining a physician's authorization, which is required by program rules. In addition, the government also alleges that, starting in 2006, some of Pacific Pulmonary Services' patient-care coordinators participated in a cross-referral kickback scheme with sleep clinics, in which they agreed to make patient referrals to sleep testing clinics in exchange for the clinics' agreement to refer patients to Pacific Pulmonary Services for sleep therapy equipment.

According to the indictment, a pulmonologist over billed for services he provided to intensive care patients at Holy Spirit Hospital. He did so from December 2007 to September 2008 by altering records kept by his employees who provided treatment to "fraudulently inflate" the time spent aiding the patients, investigators claim. The alleged fraud not only hit Medicare, but also private insurers Highmark Inc. and Capital Blue Cross. The money-laundering allegations center on claims that Clark transferred more than $100,000 of the pulmonologist's supposedly ill-gotten gains to his firm's payroll and into money-market accounts.

A Chicago pulmonologist has been identified as holding the same position at Sacred Heart Hospital as "Physician D," the doctor federal authorities' say performed medically unnecessary tracheotomies at the West Side hospital, according to a report. In a 90-page complaint released in April, federal authorities say Physician D deliberately over sedated patients, so they would not be able to breath on their own. Once a patient was deemed dependent on a ventilator, the doctor would order a tracheotomy, the complaint alleges. Physician D is described in the complaint as the chair of the critical-care committee of Sacred Heart's medical staff. Increasing numbers of troubled sleepers are seeking diagnosis and treatment of chronic sleep disorders that affect more than fifty million Americans.

The significant growth in sleep medicine over recent years brings increasing opportunities for the unscrupulous to engage in fraudulent services and billing. The most common method of diagnosing sleep disorders is a polysomnography test, which involves the monitoring and assessing of physiological reactions during sleep. Results of this test might show, for example, the presence of obstructive sleep apnea (OSA). A diagnosis of OSA often leads to a prescription for a continuous positive airway pressure (CPAP) device, which keeps the patient's airway open and unobstructed during sleep.

Medicare spending on polysomnography services is extremely high: $407 million in 2005, increasing to $565 million in 2011. With the uptick in sleep disorder services and government spending comes the discovery of various schemes that defraud federal and state health care programs that reimburse for such services.

Medicare, Medicaid, and other government programs reimburse claims for sleep tests and devices that are "reasonable and necessary" or "medically necessary" and impose a number of related requirements. For example, Medicare reimbursement requires that sleep tests be conducted by physicians or properly licensed or certified sleep technologists. Sleep tests also must be performed under the appropriate level of doctor supervision, including overall direction and control. Moreover, independent diagnostic testing facilities (e.g., non-hospital based sleep test centers), must be properly enrolled and approved by Medicare on a location-by-location basis. A provider who knowingly fails to meet these requirements yet bills a government program might be violating the False Claims Act.

Another area of potential abuse is the prescribing and dispensing of durable medical equipment (DME) such as CPAP devices. Knowingly prescribing and seeking reimbursement for devices without demonstrating the proper need defrauds government health care programs. As with independent diagnostic sleep study facilities, each location of a DME supplier must be in an appropriate site that is separately enrolled and approved by Medicare. Moreover, DME, with its individual sizing and pressure settings, must be dispensed by properly qualified personnel. Federal laws and regulations also prohibit certain self-interested dealing or business-overlap between sleep-test providers and device suppliers. The federal government repeatedly identifies fraud related to sleep testing as particularly warranting attention.

A pulmonologist, who provided critical care services to patients of a hospital, was also indicted on charges that from December 2007 through September 2008, he intentionally inflated the amount of time the health care providers he employed spent with each patient, thereby fraudulently inflating the claims he submitted to Medicare, Highmark, Inc. and Capital Blue Cross.

A Fresno County jury has awarded more than $600,000 to who said she was wrongfully terminated at a sleep medicine center because she blew the whistle on Medicare fraud. She alleged that her employer, Central California Faculty Medical Group, eliminated her position at University North Medical Specialty Center in retaliation for the fraud complaints she made and for refusing to perform medical services outside the scope of her respiratory care license.

A respiratory therapist said doctors left the responsibility to her to have in person evaluations with patients on continuous positive airway pressure, a treatment that keeps the airways open for people who have sleep apnea and other breathing problems. The patient and Medicare were later billed for a doctor's visit, even though the patient was not seen by a doctor, the lawsuit said.

Pulmonary services provide stationary and portable oxygen tanks and supplies, along with equipment for sleep therapy such as continuous-positive-airway pressure, and bi-level positive airway pressure masks, to patients in their homes. More than a dozen years ago and until the end of 2015, the Dept. of Justice alleged, a pulmonary services company submitted false claims to MediCal, Medicare, Medicaid and other federal employee-health-benefits programs for home-oxygen equipment without physician authorization. Some of the company's patient-care coordinators allegedly made patient referrals to sleep-testing clinics in exchange for those clinics referring patients to Pacific Pulmonary Services for sleep-therapy equipment. "Home oxygen equipment and related supplies are some of the most fraudulently billed items of durable medical equipment," stated a special agent in charge of the Office of Inspector General for the U.S. Department of Health and Human Services.

The former Intermune CEO is accused of creating a market for Actimmune, a medication, that reached $141 million in sales in 2003 by falsely claiming through news releases and sales campaigns that the drug substantially reduced the death rate for patients with idiopathic pulmonary fibrosis, a progressive scarring of the lungs. The drug, which cost patients $50,000 a year, actually failed to show such benefits in clinical trials, according to federal prosecutors.

Health care consumers need to identify these health care fraudsters and report them to attempt to salvage the health care system. People need to remember that he/she could receive a monetary reward for being a whistle blower.

Whistle blowers are people who expose unethical or illegal wrongdoing within companies by reporting it internally to superiors or externally to the media, government authorities, or specialized attorneys. They can be either current or past employees (insiders), or outside individuals who are familiar with the unlawful conduct, and are not required to be U.S. citizens. If you properly report Medicare fraud, you may be entitled to a significant whistleblower reward.

52. Radiology Fraud

Radiology as defined by Wikipedia is a medical specialty that uses imaging to diagnose and treat diseases seen within the body. Radiologists use a variety of imaging techniques such as X-ray radiography, ultrasound, computed tomography (CT), nuclear medicine, including positron emission tomography (PET), and magnetic resonance imaging (MRI) to diagnose and/or treat diseases.

With the slow pace of processing claims for radiology, it's a perfect place to commit fraud. Many times, it can be months or years before the government or a carrier is wise to multiple claims on behalf of the same person, or billed imaging that's never taken. Perhaps the easiest kind of fraud to identify in all of radiology is an inappropriate relationship between a referring physician and an imaging center or hospital.

For example, in the recent "Operation Ray Scam" kickback scheme in New Jersey, an imaging center bribed a physician for referrals to the benefit of both parties. Referring physicians aren't always compensated with under-the-table cash in these instances. The payoff could come in the form of a hospital working out a 'sweetheart' deal for a physician to rent out space or even a hospital handing out a high-ranking staff position.

The inspector general's office of the U.S. Department of Health and Human Services (HHS) led the raids. Those arrested are charged with taking monthly cash payments to refer Medicare and Medicaid patients to an MRI center in New Jersey. Patients have every right to expect their doctors will recommend medical service providers because they do the best job, not because they provide the best bribes.

At the end of each month, the clinic would calculate how many tests had resulted from patient referrals by each of the people arrested on Tuesday. Depending on those totals, the suspects would be paid amounts ranging from $200 to more than $5,000 per month, the release said. The U.S. attorney said that during the two months from early October through early December this year, 32 payments totaling $51,500 went from the clinic to the doctors and the nurse practitioner.

A Long Island radiology company, pleaded guilty to two counts of health care fraud for illegally performing and billing for procedures that had not been ordered by treating physicians. After accepting the guilty plea, United States District Court Judge Joanna Seybert approved a settlement with the United States and the State of New York in which the radiologist agreed to forfeit $2.4 million in the criminal case and pay $8,153,727 million to resolve civil liability arising from its fraudulent practices.

In the Tampa Bay area, was accused of submitting false claims to federal health care programs, and not observing a safety requirement that says physicians have to supervise the administration of contrast dye for an MRI. The settlement also includes accusations that the radiology center wrongly billed for procedures referred by chiropractors.

The owner of a Maryland mobile imaging provider that performed radiology studies that were allegedly never read by actual physicians has been indicted in a U.S. District Court in Baltimore.

As alleged in the complaint, in approximately May 2010, a radiologist took over the operations of a diagnostic center after the former owner, who was a radiologist, left the practice. Between May 2010 and May 2012, from his residence in Manhattan, the new radiologist and others, he employed billed Medicare and Medicaid for more than $30 million for radiological services that were not performed, using the identity of the radiologist and former owner of UMD without the doctor's knowledge or consent.

Another practice bribed that radiologist with patient referrals and received compensation for those referrals as part of an illegal scheme, the suit alleges, as part of a way to keep a "stranglehold" on its monopoly of radiology services in the community. The suit alleges that the compensation that one practice has received from an imaging center included an oversized ownership in the company, distributions from the imaging center of about $2 million a year, free services and a non-compete agreement with its employees, all of which, attorneys argue, violates the Federal Anti-Kickback Statute. And it's this scheme that resulted in millions of dollars of false or fraudulent claims paid to the hospital and imaging center by Medicare, Medicaid and other federal health care programs, the suit alleges.

United States Attorney Sally Quillian Yates said of a verdict, "This physician fraudulently cut corners at the expense of the hospitals he worked for and the patients who were being treated. He produced tens of thousands of reports claiming to include his medical findings and diagnoses based on radiology studies that had been performed, when in fact; all those interpretations had been performed by non-qualified medical assistants.

Another imaging center was forced to pay $8.71 million to the government to settle allegations that it violated the False Claims Act by billing federal health care programs for radiology procedures that patients didn't need or were rendered in an "unconscionable" way that violated federal rules for reimbursement.

Federal prosecutors said that the radiology center routinely administered injectable contrast dye into patients during MRI scans without physician supervision, as required by law because of the risk of anaphylactic shock the procedure can cause. The U.S. Department of Justice (DOJ) said that the radiology center knew of this safety requirement but "rarely, if ever, had a physician present when contrast dye was being administered."

"It is unconscionable for a physician to allow someone without the proper medical training to administer a test that could cause serious harm," said Health and Human Services Special Agent Shimon Richmond. "Not only do the kinds of frauds that were alleged in this case rob Medicare of needed funds, they threatened the health of elderly and disabled Americans."

The radiology center also performed radiology procedures that were never ordered by the patients' health care providers and then billed Medicare for the treatments when it knew that independent diagnostic testing facilities are prohibited from adding any treatments to patients without a written order from the patient's doctor. The DOJ also found the company engaged in the practice of giving kickbacks to physicians for their Medicare referrals to boost their Medicare-derived profits in violation of the Anti-Kickback Statute and Stark Law.

In a region known for health care fraud and abuse, the latest South Florida medical field to be scrutinized involves companies that have portable X-ray machines that scan patients unable to leave home, nursing homes, adult living facilities and the like. Medicare mistakenly paid the companies for X-rays that were not ordered by doctors, as federal law requires, or that were billed excessively, according to the report. Investigators urged Medicare to go after the money.

"Waste is expensive, with unnecessary imaging estimated to cost the country billions, possibly even as high as $10 billion annually," states Gregg P. Allen, M.D., executive vice president and

Chief Medical Officer of MedSolutions. "When these procedures are warranted by patient condition, they are among the best diagnostic tools available. However, procedures that are simply ordered as a result of patient demand, physician uncertainty, or lack of information that leads to repetitive and duplicative procedures, the result is the performance of unwarranted studies, with attendant unnecessary costs, and in some cases risk to the patients involved. "

The owners of two management companies allegedly illegally took $2.5 million from Allstate Corp. by controlling two radiology centers, despite not being physicians, the insurer said Wednesday in a Racketeer Influenced and Corrupt Organizations Act suit in New York federal court. The radiology centers were established so they could collect payments from the insurers of individuals in car accidents.

Soon after joining a radiology center in 2010, an employee discovered that the company regularly falsified Medicare and Medicaid claims for services rendered by uncredentialed physicians or at unenrolled practice locations. Senior executives directed her to do whatever was necessary "to get the claims paid." Despite her warnings that this constituted fraud, this individual continued to engage in its schemes. Similarly, this radiology center's executives ordered its schedulers to "split up" certain tests, i.e. schedule them on different days, no matter how inconvenient and contrary to patients' needs, because the clinic was paid more when the tests were split.

Another employee of another center complained repeatedly about improper practices, such as automatically performing pelvic and transvaginal ultrasounds an extremely invasive physical exam on female patients when their treating physicians had ordered only one of these tests.

A former chief administrator at Brooke Army Medical Center's radiology department was sentenced Friday to four years in federal prison and ordered to pay $402,485 for conspiring with a doctor who worked there to rig $8 million in military contracts.

The retired Army individual admitted in January that he and a radiologist of Kansas took advantage of rules that give preference to small, disadvantaged businesses in a scheme that involved kickbacks to the retired Army person. The two secretly steered work performed under $8.15 million in contracts to companies run by three companies and these contracts were for magnetic resonance imaging gear, staff and other services.

Recently a psychiatrist was handed a white envelope filled with $470 in cash in his West Orange office, federal authorities said Tuesday. The physiatrist was accepting a kickback reward for referring several of his patients to Orange Community MRI for diagnostic testing in October, according to those authorities.

Another physician, a board-certified radiologist and president of a teleradiology company based out of Atlanta, Georgia was arraigned this past Friday on US federal charges of wire fraud, mail fraud, healthcare fraud, and obstruction of justice. According to the federal records of the indictment, between May of 2007 and January of 2008, this doctor allegedly signed and submitted thousands of radiology reports without reviewing or interpreting the radiographs or other imaging.

Furthermore, this radiologist employed radiology physician assistants) to preview films, but they are not allowed legally to make final interpretations. Allegations state that the radiologist simply signed off on their reports without reviewing the actual images. This has affected interpretations that were provided via his company which provided tele radiology coverage to numerous hospitals in the region.

Health care consumers need to identify these health care fraudsters and report them to attempt to salvage the health care system. People need to remember that he/she could receive a monetary reward for being a whistle blower.

Whistle blowers are people who expose unethical or illegal wrongdoing within companies by reporting it internally to superiors or externally to the media, government authorities, or specialized attorneys. They can be either current or past employees (insiders), or outside individuals who are familiar with the unlawful conduct, and are not required to be U.S. citizens. If you properly report Medicare fraud, you may be entitled to a significant whistleblower reward.

53. Urology Fraud

Urology also known as genitourinary surgery is the branch of medicine that focuses on surgical and medical diseases of the male and female urinary tract system and the male reproductive organs. The organs under the domain of urology include the kidneys, adrenal glands, ureters, urinary bladder, urethra, and the male reproductive organs (testes, epididymis, vas deferens, seminal vesicles, prostate, and penis).

In Houston, a federal grand jury in May returned a three-count indictment against a urologist and his wife, charging that the doctors conspired to defraud multiple health care benefit programs, including Medicare and Medicaid and major health care insurers, from January 2003 through Feb. 24, 2012. The indictment says they submitted false and fraudulent claims in connection with the usage of unlicensed, unqualified medical personnel and billed for medical services not provided. The indictment says the practice submitted claims for urology services performed by one doctor when he was actually traveling outside the state of Texas and outside the U.S. The services were performed, according to the indictment, by medical assistants without supervision. The charges against this doctor are just an example of the government's determination to crack down on health care fraud and abuse. More headlines can be expected, and urologists may find themselves contacted as federal agents investigate everything from up coding, making false claims regarding evaluation and management services, and imaging services.

Another complaint alleges that between 2003 and 2009, a physician violated Medicare regulations by conducting medically unnecessary diagnostic tests and then seeking improper and excessive reimbursement amounts from Medicare. Moreover, the doctor was charged with submitting bills for a number of daily procedures that the Complaint alleges he was physically unable to achieve.

The settlement announced resolved allegations that scope caused to be submitted claims to Medicare and Tricare for fluorescence in situ hybridization, or "FISH," tests that were not medically necessary. FISH tests are laboratory tests performed on urine that can detect genetic abnormalities associated with bladder cancer. Medicare does not consider a FISH test reasonable or necessary unless it's used to monitor for tumor recurrence in a patient previously diagnosed with bladder cancer or unless, after performing a full work-up, the physician has reason to suspect that a patient with hematuria (i.e., blood in the urine) may have bladder cancer.

In January 2009, the doctor began referring all the FISH testing ordered by him to a laboratory owned and operated by 21st Century. He was paid bonuses by the company, based, in part, on the number of FISH tests, he referred to 21st Century laboratory. The resolution is based on the doctor's ability to compensate.

A Los Gatos doctor was sentenced Friday to a year in jail for falsely telling an 87-year-old patient he had prostate cancer and convincing him to undergo unnecessary therapy in which small radioactive rods were inserted into him with needles. This doctor was also accused of falsifying pathology reports for two other patients and recommending they undergo the treatment, known as brachytherapy. The doctor's deception was uncovered before those two men had the procedure, Santa Clara County prosecutors said. All three instances were in 2005.

An indictment alleges the urologists conspired to violate Iranian Sanctions by transferring approximately $1.1 million to Iran. The doctor allegedly utilized an unlicensed money remitting business called the Espadana Exchange to avoid the United States banking regulations and to allegedly make it appear they were not violating the United States embargo with Iran.

The indictment alleged the defendants sent some of the money representing profits of their alleged illegal health care fraud scheme to Iran for the purpose of making an investment on behalf of Hossein Lahiji and Najmeh Vahid Lahiji in real estate rental property in Iran, all in violation of the Iranian sanctions.

A laboratory company has agreed to pay $19.75 million to the government to resolve allegations that it violated the False Claims Act by billing federal health care programs for laboratory tests that were not medically necessary, the Justice Department announced today. This company is a nationwide provider of integrated cancer care services that is headquartered in Fort Myers, Florida.

A dramatic federal bust in April 2013 of a Chicago hospital and some of its physicians yielded its first prison term last week, and a light one at that a federal district judge sentenced a 74-year-old urologist to 6 months behind bars after he pleaded guilty earlier this year of receiving kickbacks for referring Medicare patients to the now-defunct hospital and bilking a private insurer for bladder tests in a separate criminal case.

Federal prosecutors sought a prison term 4 to five times that long. However, the judge may have been swayed by the defense attorney's plea for mercy for his client, whom he characterized in a court filing as an elderly "broken man in very poor physical and mental health" and a "full-blown alcoholic" who was once a good physician.

Venture of Abbott Laboratories and Takeda Chemical Industries agreed to pay $875 million to settle criminal and civil charges that it had illegally manipulated the Medicare and Medicaid programs. The settlement against the joint venture, TAP Pharmaceutical Products, is the largest for health care fraud. Prosecutors contended that sales representatives for TAP gave doctors free samples of Lupron, a drug used to treat prostate cancer and infertility, and then helped them get government reimbursements at hundreds of dollars for each dose.

Prosecutors also indicted six current and former employees of TAP charging them with conspiracy to pay kickbacks to doctors if they prescribed Lupron. The kickbacks included trips to resorts, medical equipment and money offered to the doctors as "educational grants," prosecutors said.

The U.S. Department of Health and Human Services' Office of Inspector General confirmed it is investigating another urology clinic, which is owned by urologists. The federal agency declined to discuss the details or status of the probe. A statement issued last month by the urology clinic denied wrongdoing. An attorney representing the practice, which includes 10 affiliated doctors, denied there was any investigation and refused to respond to questions.

A report last November revealed that investigators were examining the doctor's referral of patients for prostate cancer treatments at the radiation oncology center, which is co-owned by two urologists. Under federal law, a physician who refers a patient elsewhere for specialized treatment cannot receive a referral fee or collect a portion of the fee charged for that treatment. Under some circumstances, however, physicians can collect fees for treatment administered in their own offices.

Two health professionals told investigators also involves suspicions that one or more area doctors have billed for excessive and unnecessary use of many other kinds of costly medical intervention, from CT scans to needle biopsies. Allegedly, the named clinics paid kickbacks to Medicare beneficiaries and used the beneficiaries' names to bill Medicare for approximately $71 million in services that were medically unnecessary and never provided.

A urologic equipment company, which provides hospitals with lithotripsy and laser services and equipment, is accused of soliciting and receiving payments from hospitals in exchange for patient referrals. Specifically, the OIG alleged that United, and some of its physician-owners, leveraged patient referrals to obtain contract business from hospitals in Illinois, Indiana and Iowa and caused certain hospitals to submit claims for designated health services that resulted from prohibited referrals in violation of the Physician Self-Referral Law (Stark law).

An academic medical center is also accused of encouraging physicians to routinely schedule simultaneous multiple surgeries in various locations and of billing Medicare for those procedures, in defiance of a Medicare requirement that attending physicians at teaching hospitals to be present at surgeries, or at least key parts of those surgeries.

According to the suit, the software let the hospital "maximize its false billing practices by taking advantage of its remote access features to schedule attending physicians to be in multiple places at once, while continuing to bill their services as if they were actually present and personally performing the services at each place." The software includes a default function that requires physicians to document that they meet Medicare's conditions for payment, the suit alleges.

To document anesthesia services, according to the suit, the software provides only one choice for describing the level of treatment: "medically directed." As such, physicians can't choose lower-reimbursement alternatives like "medical supervision," though, the suit continues, the latter would be more accurate in almost all the medical centers cases.

Health care consumers need to identify these health care fraudsters and report them to attempt to salvage the health care system. People need to remember that he/she could receive a monetary reward for being a whistle blower.

Whistle blowers are people who expose unethical or illegal wrongdoing within companies by reporting it internally to superiors or externally to the media, government authorities, or specialized attorneys. They can be either current or past employees (insiders), or outside individuals who are familiar with the unlawful conduct, and are not required to be U.S. citizens. If you properly report Medicare fraud, you may be entitled to a significant whistleblower reward.

54. Virology Fraud

Wikipedia describes virology as the study of viruses which are submicroscopic, parasitic particles of genetic material contained in a protein coat and virus-like agents. It focuses on the following aspects of viruses: their structure, classification and evolution, their ways to infect and exploit host cells for reproduction, their interaction with host organism physiology and immunity, the diseases they cause, the techniques to isolate and culture them, and their use in research and therapy. Virology is considered to be a subfield of microbiology or of medicine.

The Food and Drug Administration has begun fighting off Internet sales of untested, unapproved flu treatments such as "generic Tamiflu" and dietary supplements that claim to prevent or treat influenza. The proliferation of these fraudulent products in online pharmacies in response to the current flu outbreak is not unexpected. In addition to Internet pharmacies, several supplement websites have been singled out for marketing flu remedies. The FDA points out that there are no legally marketed over-the-counter drugs to prevent or cure influenza, and as such, products that haven't been evaluated by the FDA but that claim to prevent or treat the flu are problematic.

At present, there are not virology medical scams reported in the news media other than the flu vaccines reported in the previous paragraph.

Health care consumers need to identify these health care fraudsters and report them to attempt to salvage the health care system. People need to remember that he/she could receive a monetary reward for being a whistle blower.

Whistle blowers are people who expose unethical or illegal wrongdoing within companies by reporting it internally to superiors or externally to the media, government authorities, or specialized attorneys. They can be either current or past employees (insiders), or outside individuals who are familiar with the unlawful conduct, and are not required to be U.S. citizens. If you properly report Medicare fraud, you may be entitled to a significant whistleblower reward.

Index

Affordable Health Care Act 25

alternative medicine 103, 104, 109, 123

ambulance fraud 51, 53, 54

chiropractic 123, 124, 125, 126, 127, 128, 150, 168, 172, 303

chronic pain 66, 71, 74, 76, 77, 82, 97, 124, 129, 149, 283, 285, 287

False Claims Act 3, 15, 17, 18, 19, 21, 22, 32, 33, 36, 43, 48, 87, 92, 114, 183, 188, 206, 237, 245, 246, 250, 251, 269, 280, 296, 297, 301, 305, 306, 316, 318, 320, 325, 330

False patient billing 1, 7

Kickbacks 9, 79, 99

Medical Identity Theft 8

medical necessity 8, 39, 40, 41, 52, 54, 90, 181, 183, 274, 305

opioid 45, 66, 67, 68, 70, 73, 74, 75, 76, 77, 78, 82, 83, 84, 85, 86, 96, 97, 141, 241

Optometry 9, 117

Phantom Billing 1, 7

Pharmaceutical company fraud 43

Pharmacy 9, 12, 21, 89, 90, 99

Pill Mill 9, 65

podiatrist 139, 140, 141, 142

topical analgesic 95

Unbundling 2, 8, 20

Up coding 2, 7, 8, 20

Upcoding fraud 20

Whistle blowers 15, 17, 19, 20, 29, 38, 49, 55, 72, 79, 88, 93, 101, 109, 115, 121, 129, 134, 138, 142, 147, 154, 161, 168, 173, 180, 186, 193, 202, 203, 206, 210, 215, 223, 229, 233, 239, 246, 254, 259, 266, 271, 278, 281, 288, 294, 298, 304, 307, 313, 321, 327, 332, 333

workers' compensation 57, 59, 60, 61, 62, 84, 92, 100, 276

About the Author

Dr. Ackerman is a clinician, academician, lecturer, author, researcher, and an expert witness in medical malpractice cases. Dr. Ackerman is: Board Certified in both Pain Medicine and Anesthesiology, is a Graduate of the University Of Louisville School Of Medicine, did a residency in anesthesiology at the University of Kentucky and was Chief Resident in Anesthesiology and Critical Care Medicine and he did a Fellowship in Pain Medicine at the Texas Tech Health Sciences Center in Lubbock, Texas.

Dr. Ackerman was: Nominated previously for the Southern Medical Society Medical Research Award, Bristol-Meyers Squibb award for distinguished achievement in Pain Research was a recipient of the Karl Koehler research grant from the American Society of Regional Anesthesia and Pain Medicine. He has been a guest speaker at medical school department meetings and academic symposiums throughout the country and at international meetings. His research has been featured in the National media.

He published sixteen books and many chapters in multiple medical textbooks including the AMA best seller: The AMA Guides to Injury and Disease Causation (First and Second editions). He authored 136 scientific articles in prestigious medical journals such as: Anesthesia Analgesia, Canadian Journal of Anaesthesia, Regional Anesthesia and Pain Management, The Journal of Hand Surgery etc.

He was a Lt. Col in the US Army and Chief of Anesthesiology of two Army medical Center Hospitals and was director of pain management at two private hospitals. Dr. Ackerman was Director of Pain Management at a University Hospital pain clinic and was an Associate Professor as well as an attending clinical instructor in critical care and hyperbaric medicine. He was director of pain management at two private hospitals and was selected to "Who's Who in International Medicine".

He is now in private practice and is president of his medical clinic. He has a strong belief in medical ethics and the prevention of medical fraud which stimulated him to write this book.

www.ingramcontent.com/pod-product-compliance
Lightning Source LLC
Chambersburg PA
CBHW020626220526
45464CB00001B/40